O9-BUB-537

THE HEALTHY
Baby Meal Planner

*Mom-Tested, Child-Approved Recipes for
Your Baby and Toddler*

ANNABEL KARMEL

Illustrations by Nadine Wickenden

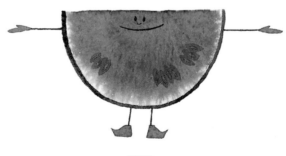

A FIRESIDE BOOK
Published by Simon & Schuster

New York   London   Toronto   Sydney

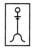

FIRESIDE
Rockefeller Center
1230 Avenue of the Americas
New York, NY 10020

Copyright © 1992, 2001, 2005 by Eddison Sadd Editions, Ltd.
Text copyright © 1992, 2001, 2005 by Annabel Karmel
All rights reserved, including the right of reproduction
in whole or in part in any form.

Revised Fireside Edition 2005

FIRESIDE and colophon are registered trademarks
of Simon & Schuster, Inc.

For information regarding special discounts for bulk purchases,
please contact Simon & Schuster Special Sales at 1-800-456-6798
or business@simonandschuster.com.

10 9 8 7 6 5 4 3 2

Library of Congress Cataloging-in-Publication Data is available.

AN EDDISON·SADD EDITION
Edited, designed, and produced by
Eddison Sadd Editions Limited
St Chad's House, 148 King's Cross Road
London WC1X 9DH
www.eddisonsadd.com

Phototypeset in Baskerville MT using
QuarkXPress on Apple Macintosh
Origination by Columbia Offset, Hong Kong
Printed in Singapore by Kyodo Printing Co Ltd

ISBN 0-7432-7404-0

*This book is dedicated
to my children,
Nicholas, Lara, and Scarlett,
and to the memory of
my first daughter,
Natasha.*

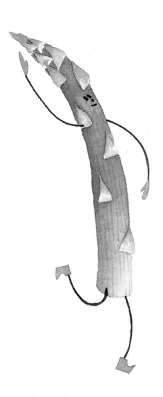

THE HEALTHY
Baby Meal Planner

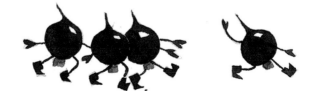

CONTENTS

ACKNOWLEDGMENTS
192

INTRODUCTION

Like any other besotted young mother, I wanted the very best for my babies. As a food lover and Cordon Bleu cook I wanted them to enjoy the wonderful tastes and aromas of fresh foods. With common sense, extensive research, two cooperative infants and a tolerant husband I knew I could create delicious recipes. Prepared quickly and easily they would be better for babies and toddlers than commercial vitamin- and iron-fortified powders and bland processed purées with a shelf life of over two years.

Poor nutrition can cause problems that will plague our children for the rest of their lives. A recent scientific study found that as many as two-thirds of cancer cases are linked to the type of food that people eat. The untimely death of my first child Natasha at the age of thirteen weeks was the catalyst that spurred me into writing this book, which has now become a valuable and popular practical guide to parents all over the world.

Battles at the dinner table are one of the more dubious pleasures of parenthood. Blessed is the mother who has never encountered the tenacious iron will of a child who will not eat. I now have three children, and the pleasure of seeing them enjoy my foods has been a wonderful experience. I am reassured to know that they are eating good fresh produce, not overprocessed convenience foods.

At a time when diet is most crucial to our child's health, why should most meals come from jars and boxes? There is no great mystique to making your own baby food, and nothing can be better than homecooked purées made from good-quality, fresh, natural ingredients. Don't be overwhelmed by the impressive lists of nutritional information on the labels of commercial baby foods; your own will contain the same goodness but without any added starches (like maltodextrin, which is the same substance that provides the glue on envelopes and stamps!).

Not only do homemade purées taste like real food, they are also much cheaper. Even busy working moms can give their baby the best start in life, since foods like mashed banana, avocado, and papaya make excellent no-cook baby purées. You can plan your baby's menus ahead and, in just two hours, prepare a whole month's food supply for your baby, freezing extra portions as purée ice cubes. You can also transform many baby purées into delicious soups for the rest of the family by adding broth and seasoning, and many meals, such as chicken casserole with vegetables, can be suitable for your baby if you set aside a portion and cook it without salt or spices.

In early childhood, eating habits and preferences (good or bad) are formed for life, so by introducing your baby to a wide range of fresh, stimulating flavors you will help establish a healthy eating pattern. Commercial carrot purées always taste the same, but with homemade purées babies get accustomed to the natural variations in the flavor of homecooked food, which helps them to adapt to family meals as they grow up.

Babies grow more rapidly in their first year than at any other time in their life. Children need calories to grow as well as an adequate supply of proteins, vitamins, and minerals. These are best provided by a healthy varied diet. Although a low-fat, high-fiber diet is fine for adults, it is not appropriate for young children. Don't be tempted to add salt or sugar to your baby's food in the first year. Salt may harm your baby's kidneys and sugar will encourage a sweet tooth – only add sugar if absolutely necessary.

If there are rules – and rules are made to be broken – they are to aim for:
• Fresh food   • Low animal fat   • Low sugar   • No added salt before one year.

A baby in the home is an opportunity to look at the dietary rules for the whole family. Some of these recipes are so delicious I serve them when entertaining! Babies' nutrition in their first year probably has greater influence than at any other time of life. This reinforces the need to start early with a good balanced diet. When your child opts for raw fruits and vegetables (which adults imagine kids hate) over sugary candy, you will recognize your success.

Good luck. I hope you and your child enjoy many happy meals together!

CHAPTER ONE

THE BEST FIRST FOODS FOR YOUR BABY

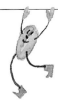

The US Department of Health and Human Services guidelines recommend breast-feeding exclusively for the first six months, as this should meet all your baby's nutritional needs. Most babies shouldn't need solid foods before the age of six months, but if you feel that your baby does need them earlier, speak to your doctor. Signs that your baby may be ready are if he is still hungry after a full milk feed, demands more frequent feeds, or wakes at night for a feed having previously slept through. There's no "right" age to introduce solids as every baby is different. However, it's important that you don't wean him too early (not before seventeen weeks) as his digestive system won't fully mature for the first few months, and foreign proteins very early on may increase the likelihood of food allergies later.

MILK IS STILL THE MAJOR FOOD

It is very important to remember when starting your baby on solids, that milk is still the best and most natural food for growing babies. I would encourage mothers to give breast-feeding a try. Apart from the emotional benefits, breast milk contains antibodies that will help protect infants from infection. In the first few months, they are particularly vulnerable and the colostrum a mother produces in the first few days of breast-feeding is a very important source of antibodies, which help to build up a baby's immune system. There are enormous benefits in breast-feeding your child, even if it is for as little as one week. It has also been medically proven that breast-fed babies are less likely to develop certain diseases in later life.

Milk should contain all the nutrients that your baby needs to grow. There are 65 calories in 4 fl oz ($^1/_2$ cup) of milk, and formula milk is fortified with vitamins and iron. Cow's milk is not such a "complete" food for human babies so is best not started until your baby is one year old. Solids are introduced to add *bulk* to a baby's diet, and to introduce new tastes, textures, and aromas; they also help the baby to practice using the muscles in his mouth. However, giving a baby too much solid food too early may lead to constipation, and provide fewer nutrients than he needs. It would be very difficult for a baby to get the equivalent amount of nutrients from the small amount of solids he will consume as he gets from his milk.

Do not use softened water or repeatedly boiled water to make your baby's bottle since they may contain concentrated mineral salts. Babies' bottles should not be warmed in a microwave, as the milk may be too hot even though the bottle feels cool to the touch. Warm the bottles by standing them in hot water.

Between four and six months babies should have 21–28 fl oz (2½–3½ cups) breast or infant formula each day. 21 fl oz (2½ cups) is enough when solids are introduced but it isn't between four and six months with no solids. It's important to make sure that, up to the age of eight months, your baby drinks milk at least four times a day (especially as it is highly likely that a bottle may not be finished at each feed). If the number of feeds is reduced too quickly, your baby will not be able to drink as much as is needed. Some mothers make the mistake of giving their baby solid food when he is hungry, when what he really needs is an additional milk feed.

Babies should be given breast or formula milk for the whole of the first year. Ordinary cow's, goat's or sheep's milk is not suitable as your baby's main drink as it does not contain enough iron and other nutrients for proper growth. However, whole cow's milk can be used in cooking or with cereal when weaning. Dairy products like yogurt and cheese can be introduced once first tastes of fruit and vegetables are accepted and are generally very popular with babies. Choose full-fat products as opposed to low-fat as babies need the calories for proper growth.

FRESH IS BEST

Fresh foods just do taste, smell, and look better than jars of pre-prepared baby foods. Nor is there any doubt that, prepared correctly, they are better for your baby (and you), for it is inevitable that nutrients, especially vitamins, are lost in the processing of preprepared baby foods. Homemade foods taste different from the jars you can buy. I believe your child will be less fussy and find the transition to joining in with family meals easier if he is used to a wide selection of fresh tastes and textures from an early age.

ORGANIC

Organic fruit and vegetables are produced without artificial chemicals, such as pesticides and fertilizers. However, there is at present no scientific evidence that pesticide levels in ordinary foods are harmful to young babies and children, but some mothers prefer not to take the risk. It is an environmentally friendly option but generates higher prices and it is up to you to decide whether it's worth the extra money.

GM FOODS

Genetic modification (GM) is the process of transferring genes from one species to another. For example, a tendency to resist frost or damage from certain insects could be implanted from one plant to another. More research needs to be done in order for us to know whether genetic modification can improve the quality and availability of crops or whether the cost to humans and the environment outweighs any benefit.

NUTRITIONAL REQUIREMENTS
Proteins

We need proteins for the growth and repair of our bodies; any extra can be used to provide energy (or is deposited as fat). Proteins are made up of different amino acids. Some foods (meat, fish, soybeans, and dairy produce including cheeses) contain all the amino acids that are essential to our bodies. Other foods (grains, legumes, nuts, and seeds) are valuable sources of protein but don't contain all the essential amino acids.

Carbohydrates

Carbohydrates and fat provide our bodies with their main sources of energy. There are two types of carbohydrate: sugar and starch (which in complex form provides fiber). In both types there are two forms – the natural and the refined. In both cases, it is the natural form of carbohydrate that provides a more healthy alternative.

SUGARS	
Natural	Fruit and fruit juices Vegetables and vegetable juices
Refined	Sugars and honey Sweetened cordials and sodas Sweet gelatins Jellies and other preserves Cakes and cookies

STARCHES	
Natural	Whole-grain breakfast cereals, flour, bread, and pasta Brown rice Potatoes Legumes, peas, and lentils Bananas and many other fruits and vegetables
Refined	Processed breakfast cereals (i.e. sugar-coated flakes) White flour, breads, and pasta White rice Sugary cookies and cakes

Fats

Fats provide the most concentrated source of energy, and babies need proportionately more fat in their diet than adults. Energy-dense foods like cheese, meat, and eggs are needed to fuel their rapid growth and development. More than 50 percent of the energy from breast milk comes from fat. Foods that contain fats also contain the fat-soluble vitamins A, D, E, and K, which arc important for the healthy development of your baby. The problem is that many people eat too much fat and the wrong type.

There are two types of fat – saturated (solid at room temperature), which mainly comes from animal sources and from artificially hardened fats found in cakes, cookies and hard margarines; and unsaturated (liquid at room temperature), which comes from vegetable sources. It is the saturated fats that are the most harmful and which may lead to high cholesterol levels and coronary disease later in life.

It is important to give your baby whole milk for at least the first two years but try to reduce fats in cooking and use butter and margarine in moderation. Try to reduce saturated fats in your child's diet by cutting down on fatty meats like fatty ground meat or sausages and replacing them with lean red meat, chicken, or oily fish.

Essential fatty acids (EFAs) are important for your baby's brain and visual development. There are two types of EFA – omega 3 from seed oils e.g.: sunflower, safflower, and corn; and omega 6 from oily fish e.g.: salmon, trout, sardines, and fresh tuna. In general we get enough omega 3 in our diets – it is the omega 6 that is often low. It is important to get the right balance of both types of EFA, especially in early life.

Vitamins

For most babies who eat fresh food in sufficient quantities and drink formula milk until the age of one year, vitamin supplements are probably unnecessary. However, the American Academy of Pediatrics recommends a daily vitamin D supplement for breast-fed infants. If your baby isn't breast-fed but drinks less than 18 fl oz (2 1/4 cups) of infant formula a day, a vitamin supplement may also be a good idea from the age of six months to two years. Ask your doctor for advice.

Children following a vegan diet should have at least 21 fl oz (2 1/2 cups) of a fortified infant soy milk daily until the age of two, then they won't need supplements. It is mainly vitamins A and D that are likely to be low in children aged six months to two years who don't have 18 fl oz (2 1/4 cups) of fortified infant or soy formula.

Vitamins are necessary for the correct development of the brain and nervous system. A good balanced diet should supply all the nutrients your child needs, and an excess of vitamins is potentially harmful, but children who are picky eaters could benefit by taking a multivitamin supplement specially designed for children.

There are two types of vitamin: water-soluble (C and B complex) and fat-soluble (A, D, E, and K). Water-soluble vitamins cannot be stored by the body, so foods containing these should be eaten daily. They can also easily be destroyed by overcooking, especially when fruit and vegetables are boiled in water. You should try to preserve these vitamins by eating the foods either raw or just lightly cooked (in a steamer, for instance).

VITAMIN A

Essential for growth, healthy skin, tooth enamel, and good vision.

Liver
Oily fish
Carrots
Dark-green leafy vegetables (e.g. broccoli)
Sweet potatoes
Squash
Tomatoes
Apricots and mangoes

VITAMIN B COMPLEX

Essential for growth, changing food into energy, maintaining a healthy nervous system, and as an aid to digestion. There are a large number of vitamins in the B group. Some are found in many foods, but no foods except for liver and yeast extract contain them all.

Meat
Sardines
Dairy produce and eggs
Whole-grain cereals
Dark-green vegetables
Yeast extract (e.g. Vegemite)
Nuts
Legumes
Bananas

VITAMIN C

Needed for growth, healthy tissue, and healing of wounds. It helps in the absorption of iron.

Vegetables such as: broccoli, bell peppers, potatoes, spinach, cauliflower.
Fruits such as: citrus fruits, blueberries, melon, papaya, strawberries, kiwi fruit.

VITAMIN D

Essential for proper bone formation, it works in conjunction with calcium. It is found in few foods, but is made by the skin in the presence of sunlight.

Oily fish
Eggs
Margarine
Dairy produce

VITAMIN E

Important for the composition of the cell structure. Helps the body create and maintain red blood cells.

Vegetable oils
Avocado
Wheatgerm
Nuts and seeds

CALCIUM

Needed for strong bones, good teeth, and growth.

Dairy products
Canned fish with bones (e.g. sardines)
Dried fruit
White bread
Green leafy vegetables and legumes

IRON

Needed for healthy blood and muscles. A deficiency in iron is probably the most common and will leave your child feeling tired and run down. Red meat is the best source of easily available iron.

Red meat, especially liver
Oily fish and egg yolks
Dried fruits (especially apricots)
Whole-grain and fortified cereals
Lentils and legumes
Green leafy vegetables

High-Risk Foods

More and more children are developing an allergy to sesame seeds, so don't give them to highly atopic babies until they're at least nine months. Berry and citrus fruits can trigger a reaction but rarely cause a true allergy. Common food allergies may cause children to feel nauseated, vomit, suffer from diarrhea, asthma, eczema, hay fever, or rashes and swelling of the eyes, lips, and face. This is one good reason why it's unwise to rush into starting your baby on solid foods.

POTENTIAL HIGH-RISK FOODS

Cow's milk and dairy produce
Nuts and seeds
Eggs
Wheat-based products
Fish (especially shellfish)
Chocolate

Water

Humans can survive for quite a time without food but only a few days without water. Babies lose more water through their kidneys and skin than adults and also through vomiting and diarrhea. Thus it's vital that they don't become dehydrated. Ensure your baby drinks plenty of fluids; cool, boiled water is the best drink to give on hot days – it's a better thirst quencher than any sugary drink. Avoid bottled mineral water as it can contain high concentrations of mineral salts, which are unsuitable for babies.

It really isn't necessary to give a very young baby anything to drink other than milk or plain water if he is just thirsty. Fruit syrups, cordials, and sweetened herbal drinks should be discouraged, to prevent dental decay. Don't be fooled if the packet says "dextrose" – this is just a type of sugar.

If your baby refuses to drink water, then give him unsweetened baby juice or fresh 100 percent fruit juices. Dilute them according to instructions, or, for fresh juice, use one part juice to three parts water.

THE QUESTION OF ALLERGIES

If your family has a history of food allergy or atopic disease such as hay fever, asthma, or eczema, there is an increased risk of developing an allergic disorder, so foods should be introduced with great care. If possible, breast-feed exclusively for the first six months. If not, discuss with your doctor the option of using a "hypoallergenic" infant formula instead. When weaning, start with low-allergen foods like baby rice, root vegetables, apple, or pear. New foods should be introduced one at a time and tried for two or three days. In that way, if there is a reaction you will know what has caused it. Avoid high-risk foods until your baby is nine to twelve months old.

There's no need to worry about food allergies unless there is a family history of allergy or atopic disease. The incidence of food allergy in normal babies is very small and, with the tendency to a later introduction of solid foods at six months, they have become even less common. Do not remove key foods like milk or wheat from your child's diet without first consulting a doctor. Although a lot of children "grow out of it" by the age of two, some allergies – particularly a sensitivity to eggs, milk, shellfish, or nuts – can last for life. If your child has an allergy, you should tell any adults who may feed him.

Never be afraid to take your baby to the doctor if you are worried. Young babies' immune systems are not fully matured and babies can become ill very quickly if they are not treated properly.

Lactose Intolerance

Lactose intolerance is not actually an allergy but the inability to digest lactose – the sugar in milk – because of a lack of a digestive enzyme. This can be hereditary, and, if this is the case, your child may experience nausea, cramps, bloating, diarrhea, and gas, usually about 30 minutes after consuming dairy foods, and should be given a special diet that avoids all dairy products. Since lactose is present in breast and cow's milk, babies who are lactose intolerant should be given soy formula. However, soy milk is not recommended for babies under the age of six months, and so these babies should be given a special low-lactose infant formula (sometimes labeled "LF").

Lactose intolerance is a rare complication that can occur after a gastrointestinal infection. In children over one year, it's safe to remove milk products for a few days to see if this makes a difference. In babies under a year, continue to breast-feed, but, if additional feeds are needed, talk to a doctor or pharmacist about using a low-lactose feed for a couple of weeks.

If a child suffers from lactose intolerance due to a lack of lactase, this will last for life.

Cow's Milk Protein Allergy

If you think your baby is sensitive to cow's milk, you should consult your doctor. Breast milk is the best alternative, but mothers should limit their own intake of dairy products as they can be transferred to their baby through breast milk. If breast-feeding has ceased, your doctor will recommend an extensively hydrolyzed (low-allergen) infant formula, which is available on prescription.

This condition means that no dairy products are tolerated. Milk-free vegetable or soy margarine may be substituted for butter. There are also many soy-based (non-dairy) yogurts and desserts available, and carob can be substituted for milk chocolate. Babies often outgrow this allergy by the age of two, but until then it is very important to ensure your child gets enough calcium in his diet.

Eggs

Eggs can be given to your baby from the age of six months but they must be cooked thoroughly until both the white and the yolk are solid. Soft-boiled eggs can be given after one year.

Fruits

Some children have an adverse reaction to citrus, berry fruits and kiwi. Rosehip or blackcurrant juice, being rich in vitamin C, make good alternatives to orange juice.

Honey

Honey should not be given to children under 12 months as it can cause infant botulism. Although this is very rare, it is best to be safe as a baby's digestive system is too immature to deal with the bug.

Nuts

It is rare to be allergic to tree nuts such as walnuts and hazelnuts. However, peanuts and peanut products can induce a severe allergic reaction – anaphylactic shock – which can be life threatening, so it's best to be cautious. In families with a history of any allergy including hay fever, eczema, and asthma, it's advisable to avoid all products containing peanuts, including peanut oil, until the child is three years old, and then seek medical advice before introducing them into the diet. Peanut butter and finely ground nuts, however, can be introduced from six months, provided there is no family history of allergy.

It is important only to buy packaged food that is labeled "nut free"; loose bakery products, candy, and chocolates may contain nuts. Children under the age of five shouldn't be given whole nuts because of the risk of choking.

Gluten

Gluten is found in wheat, rye, barley, and oats. Foods containing gluten, such as bread or pasta, should not be introduced into any baby's diet before six months.

When buying baby cereals and teething biscuits, choose varieties that are gluten free. Baby rice is the safest to try at first, and thereafter there are plenty of alternative gluten-free products such as soy, corn, rice, millet, rice noodles, and buckwheat spaghetti, and potato flours for thickening and baking.

In some cases, intolerance to wheat and similar proteins is temporary, and children may grow out of the condition before they are two or three years old. However, although it is rare, some people suffer from a permanent sensitivity to gluten known as celiac disease. Symptoms include loss of appetite, poor growth, swollen abdomen, and pale and particularly smelly stools. Celiac disease can be diagnosed by a blood test and can be confirmed by looking at the gut wall using endoscopy.

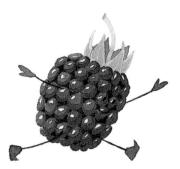

PREPARING BABY FOODS

Preparing and cooking baby foods isn't difficult, but, because you're dealing with a baby, considerations like hygiene must be of the utmost importance. Always wash fruit and vegetables carefully before cooking.

Equipment

You will already have most of the equipment you need – mashers, graters, strainers, etc. – but the following pieces you may not, and I consider them to be vital!

Food mill A hand-turned mill or ricer with variable cutting discs purées the food and removes seeds and skin which can be difficult for a baby to digest. It is ideal for dried apricots, corn, and green beans.

Blender or food processor This is useful for puréeing larger quantities. However, foods for young babies will often need to be pushed through a strainer afterwards to remove any indigestible seeds and skin.

Steamer It is worth buying a good multi-tiered steamer that will enable you to cook several different foods at the same time. (A colander placed over a saucepan, with a well-fitting lid, is a cheaper alternative.)

Sterilizing

At first, it is very important to sterilize bottles properly, and particularly the teats that your baby sucks, by whatever approved method you choose. Warm milk is the perfect breeding ground for bacteria and, if bottles are not properly washed and sterilized, your baby can become very ill. It would be impossible, however, to sterilize *all* the equipment you use for cooking and puréeing baby food, but take extra care to keep everything very clean.

Use a dishwasher if you have one; the water is at a much higher temperature than it would be possible to use if washing the utensils by hand, which helps to sterilize your equipment. However, once it is removed from the dishwasher, it does not remain sterile; bottles should be filled with milk immediately and stored in the refrigerator. Dry utensils with paper towels rather than a non-sterile dish towel.

All milk bottles should continue to be sterilized until your baby is one year old, but there is really not much point in sterilizing spoons or food containers beyond the age when your baby starts to crawl and put everything in reach into his mouth. There is no need to sterilize any other feeding equipment, but do wash bowls and spoons in a dishwasher or by hand at about 80°F – you will need to wear rubber gloves. If using a food processor, it is a good idea to rinse it out with boiling water as they are a common breeding ground for bugs.

Steaming

Steam the vegetables or fruits until tender. This is the best way to preserve the vitamins and fresh flavor. Vitamins B and C are water soluble and can easily be destroyed by overcooking, especially when foods are boiled in water. Broccoli loses over 60 percent of its antioxidants when boiled, but less than 7 percent when steamed.

Boiling

Peel, seed, or pit the vegetables or fruits as necessary and cut into pieces. Try to use the minimum amount of water and be careful not to overcook. To make a smooth purée, add a small amount of the cooking liquid, or formula or breast milk.

Microwaving

Place the vegetables or fruits in a suitable dish. Add a little water, cover leaving an air vent, and cook on full power until tender (stir halfway through). Purée to the desired consistency. Check that it isn't too hot for your baby and stir well to avoid hot spots.

Baking

If you are cooking a meal for the family in the oven, you could use the opportunity to bake a potato, sweet potato or butternut squash for your baby. Prick the chosen vegetable with a fork and bake until tender. Cut in half (remove the seeds from the squash), scoop out the flesh and mash together with some water or milk.

Freezing Baby Foods

Preparing tiny amounts of purée can be difficult. It is much better to prepare more than you need and freeze extra portions in ice-cube trays or small pots. You can then plan your baby's meals so that you only need to cook once or twice a week.

Cook and purée the food, cover and cool as quickly as possible. To preserve the quality of the food, it is very important that any foods that are to be frozen are well sealed to prevent the food drying out. It is also best if the container is filled almost to the top rather than leaving a large pocket of air above the food. It should be stored in a freezer that will freeze food to 0°F or below in 24 hours.

In the early stages of weaning, flexible plastic ice-cube trays are ideal for freezing baby food, but make sure you wrap them

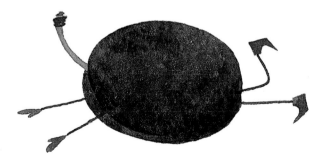

in plastic freezer bags. Once frozen, knock the cubes out and store them in freezer bags, labeling them with the expiration date so you never give food that is past its best. Squeeze out as much air as possible before sealing securely, in order to maximize storage life. Once your baby starts eating larger portions, it is a good idea to buy some small, plastic containers with snap-on lids that are designed for freezing baby food.

To thaw one meal, remove the relevant number of cubes from the bag (if there is time, leave the food to defrost before heating) and heat in a small pan or a microwave until piping hot all the way through (stir thoroughly if heating in a microwave). Allow the food to cool down and always test the temperature before feeding your baby as their mouths are more sensitive to heat than ours. Fruit that is to be served cold can be defrosted in the refrigerator overnight. There are some rules regarding frozen food.

- Never refreeze meals that have already been frozen; however, if using frozen vegetables or fruit to make baby purées they can be cooked and refrozen.
- Never reheat meals more than once.
- Baby foods can be stored in a freezer for up to 8 weeks.

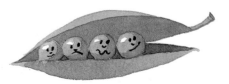

INTRODUCING PARTICULAR FOODS

I have listed below particular foods that you should avoid feeding your baby until a certain age has been reached. This is not an exhaustive list and you should refer to each chapter for more information.

WHEN CAN THEY HAVE ...?	
Gluten (wheat, rye, barley and oats)	6 months
Citrus fruits	6 months
Well-cooked eggs	6–9 months
Soft eggs, e.g. well-cooked scrambled eggs	from 1 year
Added salt	limited amount from 12 months
Sugar	limited amount from 12 months
Whole cow's milk as a main drink	12 months
Honey	12 months
Paté	12 months
Soft/blue cheese e.g. Brie/Gorgonzola	12 months
Whole/chopped nuts	5 years

MEAL PLANNERS

In the next chapter I've devised some meal planners to help you through the first weeks when you start to wean your baby. The First Tastes Meal Planner shows how to gradually wean your baby onto solids using mainly single-ingredient, easily digested fruit and vegetable purées that are unlikely to provoke an allergic reaction. Once your baby has been introduced to these tastes, progress to the After First Tastes Accepted Meal Planner, which includes combinations of fruit and vegetable purées like carrot and pea, or peaches, apples, and pears. Adapt the recipes according to what is in season.

These planners are intended only as a guide and will depend on many factors including weight. If your baby's last meal is close to bedtime, avoid giving him anything that is heavy or difficult to digest. This is certainly not the time to experiment with new foods if you both want a good night's sleep.

I have tried to give a wide choice of recipes, although I expect that meals your baby enjoys will be repeated several times – and this is where your freezer is useful.

In each subsequent chapter, there are meal planners for your baby that you may follow or simply use as a guide. Adapt the charts according to what's in season and what you're preparing for your family. From nine months onwards, you should be able to cook for your baby and family together, perhaps eating the recipes you give your baby

for lunch and supper for your own supper, provided you do not add salt to your baby's portion.

In these later charts, I have set out four meals a day, but many babies will be satisfied with three meals as well as some healthy snacks.

Many of the vegetable purées in the early chapters can be transformed into a vegetable soup, and a number of the vegetable dishes can serve as good side dishes for the family. Again, if you give the baby some of the vegetables you are preparing for the family, make sure you haven't added salt. In the later chapters many recipes are suitable for the whole family.

After each recipe is a symbol of two faces – one smiling ☺, the other gloomy ☹ – each with a tick box. You will find these useful for recording your successes (or otherwise)! Some recipes also show a snowflake ✳, which means the meal is suitable for freezing.

CHAPTER TWO

FIRST-STAGE WEANING

In the recent past there was a lot of pressure on parents to start their babies on solids too early – this pressure was variously commercial, medical, and social (keeping up with the neighbor's baby!). Ideas have now changed, and this is all to the good, for many ordinary foods, as already discussed, can cause allergies. Neither is a baby's digestive system capable of absorbing foods more complex than baby milk until the age of at least seventeen weeks.

The US Department of Health and Human Services guidelines recommend breast-feeding exclusively for the first six months as that should meet all your baby's nutritional needs. If a baby is being given formula milk she will need 21–28 fl oz (2½–3½ cups) a day between four and six months, and 18–28 fl oz (2¼–3½ cups) a day between six months and one year once she starts on solids.

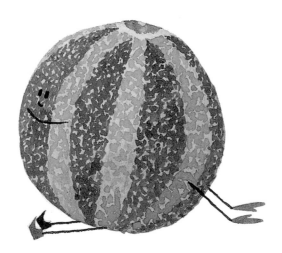

FIRST FRUITS AND VEGETABLES

Very first foods should be easy to digest and unlikely to provoke an allergic reaction.

I find that root vegetables like carrot, sweet potato, parsnip, and rutabaga tend to be the most popular with very young babies due to their naturally sweet flavor and smooth texture once puréed. The best first fruits for young babies are apple, pear, banana, and papaya, but it's important that you choose fruit that is ripe and has a good flavor, so it's a good idea to taste it yourself before giving it to your baby.

Until recently, the advice given was to introduce each food separately, waiting for three days before introducing another new food. However, unless there is a history of allergy or you are concerned about your baby's reactions to a certain food, there is no reason why new foods should not be introduced on consecutive days, provided you keep to the list in the table.

Take care when introducing solids *not to reduce your baby's milk intake*, as milk is still the most important factor in growth and development.

It is important to wean your baby on as wide a range of foods as possible. After first tastes are accepted you can introduce all fruit and vegetables (see page 27). However, take care with citrus, pineapple, berry fruits and kiwi fruit as these may upset some susceptible babies.

BEST FIRST FRUITS

Apple
Pear
Banana*
Papaya*

BEST FIRST VEGETABLES

Carrot
Potato
Rutabaga
Parsnip
Pumpkin
Butternut squash
Sweet potato

* Banana and papaya do not require cooking provided they are ripe. They can be puréed or mashed on their own or together with a little breast or formula milk. Bananas are not suitable for freezing.

Fruit

At first a baby should have cooked purées of fruits like apple and pear, or uncooked, mashed banana or papaya. After a few weeks your baby can graduate to other raw, mashed or puréed fruits like melon, peach and plum – these are delicious when ripe.

Dried fruits can be introduced but in small quantities; although they are nutritious they tend to be laxatives. If you are worried about the use of pesticides, organic fruit and vegetables are available.

Vegetables

Some people prefer to start their babies on vegetables rather than fruit. Because most babies will take to eating fruit quite

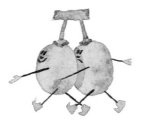

happily, they feel it is important to establish a liking for more savory tastes.

At the beginning, when introducing a baby to solids, it is best to start with root vegetables, particularly carrots, since they are naturally sweet. Different vegetables provide different vitamins and minerals (for instance, green vegetables provide vitamin C, and yellow provide vitamin A) so a variety is of value at later stages.

Many vegetables have quite strong flavors – broccoli, for instance – so when solids are fairly well established, you could mix in some potato or baby rice and milk to make them more palatable. Very young babies like their food quite bland.

Note that all fruits and vegetables can also be cooked in a microwave (see page 17 for general method).

Rice

Another good first food is baby rice. Mixed with water, breast, or formula milk, it is easily digested and its milky flavor makes for a smooth transition to solids. Choose one that is sugar free and enriched with vitamins and iron. Baby rice also combines well with both fruit and vegetable purées.

TEXTURES

At the very beginning of weaning, the rice and fruit or vegetable purées should be fairly wet and soft. This means that most vegetables should be cooked until very soft so that they purée easily. You may need to thin out the consistency of the purées since babies are more likely to accept food in a semi-liquid form. To do this, you can use formula or breast milk, fruit juice, or some boiled water.

As your baby gets used to the feel of "solid food" in her mouth, you can gradually reduce the amount of liquid that you add to purées, which will encourage her to chew a little. This should be a natural process as she should want to chew her food as she starts teething (this usually occurs between six and twelve months). You could also *thicken* the purées if necessary with some baby rice or crumbled rusk. As your baby becomes older and solid feeding is established (at about six months), some fruit can be served raw and vegetables cooked more lightly (thereby retaining more vitamin C). Food can also be mashed or finely chopped to encourage chewing later on.

Remember to peel, core, and seed fruits as necessary before cooking and/or puréeing them (or put them through a food mill). Vegetables with fibers or seeds should be strained or put through a food mill for a smooth texture. The husks of leguminous vegetables cannot be digested by a baby at this stage.

QUANTITIES

At the very beginning, don't expect your baby to take more than 1–2 teaspoons of her baby rice or a fruit or vegetable purée. For this you should need one portion – in this section, this means one or two cubes from an ice-cube tray.

As your baby gets used to eating solids you may need to defrost three or more frozen food-cubes for her meal, or start freezing food in larger pots.

DRINKS

Water, as outlined on page 13, is the best drink to offer. However, freshly squeezed orange juice is high in vitamin C, which helps your child to absorb iron. If your baby reacts to orange juice, you can offer blackcurrant or rosehip instead. Dilute one part juice to at least five parts cooled boiled water. Diluted juice tastes weak to us but babies don't miss the sweet taste as they haven't been used to it. Try to avoid giving sweet drinks as this will give them a sweet tooth and will result in them no longer accepting water.

If you buy commercial fruit juices, they should be unsweetened. But, even those labeled "unsweetened" or "no added sugar" still contain sugars and acids that can lead to tooth decay. It is important not to let your baby continually sip any fluid except water.

A juicer is a useful appliance to have at home. Many fruits *and* vegetables can be turned into nutritious drinks.

TIPS FOR INTRODUCING SOLIDS

1 Make the rice or purée fairly wet and soft at first, using breast or formula milk, an unsweetened juice, or cooking water. A handy tip is to mix the purée in the plastic removable top of a feeding bottle (which has been sterilized).

2 Hold your baby comfortably on your lap or sit her in her baby chair. It would be better if *both* of you were protected against spills!

3 Choose a time when your baby is not frantically hungry and maybe give her some milk first to partially satisfy her – she will then be more receptive to the new idea.

4 Babies are unable to lick food off a spoon with their tongues, so choose a small, *shallow* plastic teaspoon off which she can take some food with her lips. (Special feeding spoons can be bought.)

5 Start by giving just one solid feed during the day, about 1–2 teaspoons to begin with. I prefer to give this feed at lunchtime.

FRUIT AND VEGETABLES

FIRST TASTES

Apple

Choose a sweet variety of dessert apple. Peel, halve, core, and chop 2 medium apples. Put into a heavy pan with 4–5 tablespoons water. Cover and cook over a low heat until tender (7–8 minutes). Or, steam for the same length of time. Purée. If steaming, add some of the boiled water from the bottom of the steamer to thin out the purée.

Apple and Cinnamon

Simmer 2 dessert apples in apple juice with a cinnamon stick. Cook as above; remove stick before puréeing.

MAKES 5 PORTIONS

Pear

Peel, halve, and core 2 pears, then cut into small pieces. Cover with a little water and cook over a low heat until soft (about 4 minutes). Or steam for the same length of time. Purée. After the first few weeks of weaning, you can purée ripe pears without cooking. Apple and pear together makes a good combination.

MAKES 5 PORTIONS

Banana

Mashed banana makes ideal baby food. It is easy to digest and rarely causes allergic reactions. Choose a small, ripe banana and mash well with a fork to make it as smooth as possible. Add a little boiled water or baby milk if it is too thick and sticky for your baby to swallow.

If your baby is suffering from diarrhea or a stomach upset, a diet of mashed banana, cooked apple purée and baby rice for a few days is a good remedy.

MAKES 1 PORTION

Papaya

Papaya is an excellent fruit to give to a very young baby. It has a pleasing, sweet taste that is not too strong and blends within seconds to a perfect texture. Ripe fruit has a yellowish skin.

Cut a medium papaya in half, remove all the black seeds, and scoop out the flesh. Purée, adding a little formula or breast milk if you like.

MAKES 4 PORTIONS

Cream of Fruit

Combining a fruit purée with baby milk and baby rice or crumbled rusk can make it more palatable for your baby. In the next few months, when your baby may start eating some other exotic fruits like mango and kiwi, this method of "diluting" the fruit purées with milk will make them less acidic.

Peel, core, steam, or boil and purée the fruit of your choice as described and, for each 4-portion quantity of prepared fruit, you should stir in 1 tablespoon unflavored baby rice or half a low-sugar rusk and 2 tablespoons baby milk.

MAKES 3 EXTRA PORTIONS

Three-Fruit Purée

This is a delicious combination of three of the first fruits that your baby can eat.

Mix 2 teaspoons each of pear and apple purées (see page 24) with half a banana, mashed. You could also use half a raw, ripe pear, peeled, cored, and cut into chunks. Purée this and the half banana in a blender until smooth, then mix together with the 2 teaspoons of cooked apple purée.

MAKES 4 PORTIONS

Carrot or Parsnip

Peel, trim, and slice 2 medium carrots or parsnips. Place in a pan of lightly boiling water, cover, and simmer for 25 minutes or until very tender. Alternately, you can steam them. Drain, reserving the cooking liquid, and purée to a smooth consistency, adding as much of the reserved liquid as necessary.

The cooking time is longer for small babies. Once your baby can chew, cut the time down to preserve the vitamin C and keep the vegetables more crisp.

MAKES 4 PORTIONS

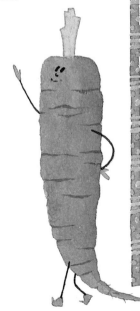

Sweet Potato, Rutabaga, or Parsnip

Use a large sweet potato, a small rutabaga, or 2 large parsnips. Scrub, peel, and chop into small cubes. Cover with boiling water and simmer, covered, until tender (15–20 minutes). Alternately, steam the vegetables. Drain, reserving the cooking liquid. Purée in a blender, adding some liquid if necessary.

MAKES 4 PORTIONS

Potato

Wash, peel and chop 14 oz potato, just cover with boiling water, and cook over a medium heat for about 15 minutes. Blend with some cooking liquid or baby milk to make the desired consistency. Alternately, steam the potato and blend with some water from the steamer or your baby's usual milk.

Avoid using a food processor to purée potato as it breaks down the starch and makes a sticky pulp. Use a food mill instead.

You can bake potatoes or sweet potatoes in the oven. Preheat to 400°F for 1–1¼ hours or until soft. Scoop out the inside and mash with a little baby milk and butter.

MAKES 10 PORTIONS

Cream of Carrot

A creamy purée can be made with many different vegetables by adding milk and baby rice. Make a purée with 1 large carrot (approx. 3 oz). This should make a scant ½ cup carrot purée (see page 25). Mix 1 tablespoon unflavored baby rice with 2 tablespoons of your baby's usual milk. Stir the baby-rice mixture into the vegetable purée. Half a low-sugar rusk crushed and mixed with baby milk will also make a creamy purée. Allow the rusk to soften in the baby milk before mixing it into the vegetable purée of your choice.

MAKES 2 PORTIONS

Butternut Squash

Butternut squash has a naturally sweet flavor that is very popular with babies.

Peel a butternut squash, weighing about 12 oz. Remove seeds and cut the flesh into 1-inch cubes. Steam or cover with boiling water and simmer for about 15 minutes or until tender. Transfer the squash to a blender and make a purée with a little of the cooking liquid.

MAKES 6 PORTIONS

FRUIT AND VEGETABLES

AFTER FIRST TASTES ACCEPTED

Zucchini

Wash 2 medium zucchini carefully, remove the ends, and slice. (The skin is soft, so doesn't need to be removed.) Steam until tender (about 10 minutes), then purée in a blender or mash with a fork. (No need to add extra liquid.) Good mixed with sweet potato, carrot, or baby rice.

MAKES 8 PORTIONS

Broccoli and Cauliflower

Use 1 cup of either. Wash well, cut into small florets, and then add $5/8$ cup boiling water. Simmer, covered, until tender (about 10 minutes). Drain, reserving the cooking liquid. Purée until smooth, adding a little of the liquid, or baby milk, to make the desired consistency.

Alternately, steam the florets for 10 minutes for better flavor and retention of nutrients. Add water from the steamer, or baby milk, to make a smooth purée. Broccoli and cauliflower are good mixed with a cheese sauce or root-vegetable purée like carrot or sweet potato.

MAKES 4 PORTIONS

Green Beans

Any variety of green bean is suitable but smaller, younger beans are more tender. Trim the beans and remove any stringy bits. Steam until tender (about 12 minutes), then blend. Add a little boiled water or baby milk to make a smooth purée. Green vegetables like beans are good mixed with root vegetables such as sweet potato or carrot.

Potato, Zucchini, and Broccoli

Combining potato with green vegetables makes it more palatable for your baby. Peel and chop 2 medium potatoes (7 oz). Boil them in water below a steamer for about 10 minutes or until soft. Place $1/4$ cup broccoli florets and $1/2$ cup sliced zucchini in the steamer basket, cover, and cook for 5 minutes or until all the vegetables are tender. Drain the potatoes and purée in a food mill with the other vegetables, adding enough baby milk to make a smooth consistency.

MAKES 4 PORTIONS

Broccoli Trio

Peel and chop a medium sweet potato (approx. 7 oz) and boil for 5 minutes. Place $1/2$ cup each of broccoli and cauliflower florets in a steamer basket above the sweet potato, cover, and continue to cook for 5 minutes. When all the vegetables are tender, purée them in a blender together with a little butter and enough of the cooking liquid to make the desired consistency.

MAKES 4 PORTIONS

Peach

Bring a small saucepan of water to a boil. Cut a shallow cross on the skin of 2 peaches, submerge them in the water for 1 minute, then plunge into cold water. Skin and chop the peaches, discarding the pits. Either purée the peaches uncooked or steam first for a few minutes until tender. Peach and banana makes a good combination.

MAKES 4 PORTIONS

Carrot and Cauliflower

Combining vegetables makes them more interesting and, once your baby has got used to carrot and cauliflower separately, this combination will make a nice change. Cook $1/2$ cup carrot, scraped and sliced, in boiling water for 20 minutes until soft. After 10 minutes, add $1 1/2$ cups cauliflower florets. Drain the vegetables and purée in a blender. Stir in 2 tablespoons baby milk.

MAKES 4 PORTIONS

Cantaloupe Melon

Cantaloupes are the small, very pale, green melons with orange flesh. They are rich in vitamins A and C. Only give ripe melon. Cut in half, remove the seeds, scoop out the flesh, and purée in a blender.

Other varieties of sweet melon like Galia or Honeydew are good too. When your baby is a little older, properly ripe melon may be eaten raw.

MAKES 6 PORTIONS

Plum

Skin 2 large ripe plums as for peaches (see opposite). Purée in a blender – the fruit can be puréed uncooked if soft and juicy, or you could steam the plums for a few minutes until tender. Plums are good mixed with baby rice, banana, or yogurt.

MAKES 4 PORTIONS

Dried Apricot, Peach, or Prune

Many grocery stores sell a selection of ready-to-eat dried fruits. Dried apricots are particularly nutritious, being rich in beta-carotene and iron. Cover $^3/_4$ cup fruit with cold water, bring to a boil, and simmer until soft (about 5 minutes). Drain, remove the pits, and pass through a mill to remove the skins. Add a little of the cooking liquid to make a smooth purée.

This is good combined with baby rice and milk, banana, or ripe pear.

MAKES 4 PORTIONS

Apricot and Pear

Roughly chop $^1/_2$ cup ready-to-eat dried apricots and put them into a saucepan with 2 ripe pears (12 oz) peeled, cored, and cut into pieces. Cook, covered, over a low heat for 3–4 minutes. Purée in a blender. Alternately, use 4 fresh, sweet, ripe apricots, peeled, pitted, and chopped.

MAKES 8 PORTIONS

Apple and Raisin Compote

Heat 3 tablespoons of fresh orange juice in a saucepan. Add 2 dessert apples peeled, cored, and sliced, and $1^1/_2$ tablespoons washed raisins. Cook gently for about 5 minutes until soft, adding a little water if necessary.

Dried fruit like apricots or raisins should be put through a food mill for young babies, to get rid of the outer skin, which is difficult to digest.

MAKES 8 PORTIONS

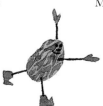

Peas

I tend to use frozen peas as they are just as nutritious as fresh. Cover 1 cup peas with water, bring to a boil, and simmer, covered, for 4 minutes. Drain, reserving some cooking liquid. Put the peas through a mill or a strainer and add a little cooking liquid to make the desired consistency. Good combined with potato, sweet potato, parsnip, or carrot. If using fresh peas, cook for 12–15 minutes.

MAKES 4 PORTIONS

Red Bell Pepper

Wash, core, and seed a medium bell pepper. Cut into quarters and roast under a preheated broiler until the skin is charred. Place in a plastic bag and let cool. Peel off the blistered skin, and purée. Good with cauliflower or potato.

MAKES 2–3 PORTIONS

Avocado

Choose a well-ripened avocado, cut it in half, and scoop out the pit. Use $^{1}/_{3}$–$^{1}/_{2}$ of the avocado and mash the flesh with a fork, maybe adding a little milk. Serve quickly, otherwise it will turn brown. Good mixed with mashed banana.

Do not freeze avocados.

MAKES 1 PORTION

Corncob

Remove the outer corn husks and silk from the corncob and rinse well. Cover with boiling water and cook over a medium heat for 10 minutes. Strain and then remove the kernels of corn using a sharp knife. Purée in a mill. Alternately, cook some frozen corn kernels and then purée.

MAKES 2 PORTIONS

Spinach

Wash 2 cups spinach leaves very carefully, removing the coarse stalks. Either steam the spinach or put in a saucepan and sprinkle with a little water. Cook until the leaves are wilted (about 3–4 minutes). Gently press out any excess water. Good combined with potato, sweet potato, or butternut squash.

MAKES 2 PORTIONS

Tomatoes

Plunge 2 medium tomatoes into boiling water for 30 seconds. Transfer to cold water, skin, seed, and roughly chop. Melt a little butter in a heavy-based pan and sauté the tomato until mushy. Purée in a blender. This is good combined with potato, cauliflower, or zucchini.

MAKES 2–3 PORTIONS

Peach and Banana

This is a delicious purée to make when peaches are in season. They are a good source of vitamin C and are easy to digest. Banana also combines well with papaya.

MAKES 1 PORTION

1 ripe peach, skinned and cut into pieces　*½ tablespoon pure apple juice*
1 small banana, peeled and sliced　*baby rice (optional)*

Put the peach, banana, and apple juice into a small pan, cover, and simmer for 2–3 minutes. Purée in a blender. If it's too runny, add a little baby rice.

Apple and Banana with Orange Juice

This makes a nice change from plain, mashed banana or apple purée. When your baby is six months or older, you can make this with raw, grated apple and mashed banana.

MAKES 1 PORTION

¼ apple, peeled, cored, and chopped　*1 teaspoon orange juice*
¼ banana, peeled and chopped

Steam the apple until tender (about 7 minutes), then purée or mash it together with the banana and orange juice. Serve as soon as possible.

Peaches, Apples, and Pears

When peaches aren't in season you can make this just using apples and pears. If the purée is too thin, stir in some baby rice to thicken it.

MAKES 8 PORTIONS

2 dessert apples, peeled, cored, and chopped
1 vanilla bean

2 tablespoons apple juice or water
2 ripe peaches, skinned and chopped
2 ripe pears, peeled, cored, and chopped

Put the chopped apple in a saucepan. Split the vanilla bean with a sharp knife, scrape the seeds into the pan, and add the bean and the apple juice or water. Simmer, covered, for about 5 minutes. Add the peaches and pears and cook for 3–4 minutes more. Remove the bean and purée.

Mixed Dried-Fruit Compote

Dried fruits and fresh fruits are delicious combined. Later on, mix with a little plain yogurt.

MAKES 6 PORTIONS

1/2 cup each of dried apricots, dried peaches, and prunes

1 dessert apple and 1 pear, peeled, cored, and chopped, or 1 apple and 3 fresh apricots, skinned, pitted, and chopped

Put the dried fruit, apple, and pear (or apricot, if using) into a saucepan, and just cover with boiling water. Simmer for about 8 minutes. Drain the fruit, and purée, adding a little of the cooking liquid if necessary.

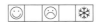

Vegetable Broth

Vegetable broth forms the basis of many vegetable recipes. This should keep for a week in the refrigerator, and it is well worth making your own, which will be free from additives and salt.

MAKES ABOUT 4 CUPS

1 large onion, peeled
4½ oz carrot, peeled
1 celery stalk
1½ cups mixed root vegetables (sweet potato, rutabaga, parsnip), peeled
½ leek

2 tablespoons butter
1 sachet bouquet garni
1 sprig of fresh parsley
1 bay leaf
6 black peppercorns
3¾ cups water

Chop all the vegetables. Melt the butter in a large saucepan and sauté the onion for 5 minutes. Add the remaining ingredients and cover with the water. Bring to a boil and simmer for about 1 hour. Strain the broth and squeeze out any remaining juices from the vegetables through a strainer.

Carrot and Pea Purée

Both carrots and peas have a naturally sweet taste that appeals to babies.

MAKES 2 PORTIONS

7 oz carrot, peeled and sliced

⅓ cup frozen peas

Put the sliced carrot in a saucepan and cover with boiling water. Cook, covered, for 15 minutes. Add the peas and cook for a further 5 minutes. Purée with sufficient cooking liquid to make a smooth purée.

Baby Cereal and Vegetables

Sometimes vegetable purées can be very watery – particularly those made from, say, zucchini which have a high water content. In this recipe I have added baby rice, which makes an excellent thickening agent.

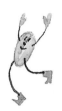

MAKES 6 PORTIONS

2 tablespoons onion, chopped
1 teaspoon olive oil
1 medium zucchini, trimmed and sliced
1/2 cup broccoli

2 medium carrots, peeled and sliced
vegetable broth (optional)
1/2 cup frozen peas
3 tablespoons baby rice

Sauté the onion in the olive oil for 2 minutes, then add all the vegetables except the frozen peas. Just cover with boiling water or vegetable broth. Bring back to a boil, then simmer for 20 minutes. Add the frozen peas and cook for 5 minutes more. Purée the vegetables, adding as much of the cooking liquid as necessary to make the desired consistency, and stir in the baby rice.

Sweet Vegetable Medley

Root vegetables, such as rutabaga, carrot, and parsnip make delicious and nutritious purées for young babies. Butternut squash and pumpkin can also be used to make this purée as, again, they are very popular with babies.

MAKES 5 PORTIONS

1 cup carrot, peeled and chopped
1 cup rutabaga, peeled and chopped
1 cup potato, butternut squash, or pumpkin, peeled and chopped

1/2 cup parsnip, peeled and chopped
1 1/4 cups water or milk (you can use cow's milk in cooking from 6 months)

Put the vegetables in a pan with the water or milk. Bring to a boil, then cover and simmer for 25–30 minutes or until the vegetables are tender. Remove with a slotted spoon and purée the vegetables in a blender, with sufficient cooking liquid to make the desired consistency.

Watercress, Potato, and Zucchini Purée

Watercress is rich in calcium and iron. It blends well with the other vegetables to make a tasty, bright green purée. You can add a little milk if your baby prefers it that way.

MAKES 6 PORTIONS

1 large potato (approx. 11 oz), peeled and chopped
1¼ cups vegetable broth (see page 33)

1 medium zucchini (approx. 4 oz), trimmed and sliced
a small bunch of watercress
a little milk (optional)

Put the potato into a saucepan, cover with the broth, and cook for 5 minutes. Add the sliced zucchini and continue to cook for another 5 minutes. Trim the stalks of the watercress, add to the potato, and cook for 2–3 minutes. Purée the mixture in a mill and, if you like, add a little milk to adjust the consistency.

Avocado and Banana or Papaya

This is very simple to make and the fruits blend very well.

MAKES 1 PORTION

½ small avocado   *½ small banana or ¼ papaya*

Remove the flesh from the avocado and mash with the banana or papaya until smooth. This should be eaten soon after it is made or the avocado will turn brown.

Butternut Squash and Pear

Butternut squash is rich in antioxidants, which help protect against cancer and boost your child's immune system. It is easily digested, rarely causes allergies, and is a good source of vitamin A, important for healthy skin and vision. Babies like its naturally sweet taste, which combines well with fruit; and cooking fruit and vegetables in a steamer, as here, is one of the best ways of preserving nutrients. Butternut squash is also delicious if you cut it in half, scoop out the seeds, brush each half with melted butter, and spoon 1 tablespoon of fresh orange juice into each cavity. Cover with foil and bake in the oven at 350°F for 1½ hours or until tender.

MAKES 4 PORTIONS

1 medium butternut squash or pumpkin   *1 ripe, juicy pear*
(about 1 lb)

Peel the butternut squash, cut in half, remove the seeds, and chop into pieces. Steam for about 12 minutes. Peel, core, and chop the pear, add to the steamer, and continue to cook for 5 minutes or until the squash is tender. Purée in a blender.

Sweet Potato with Cinnamon

The addition of cinnamon gives this an extra sweetness, which babies love. This is very simple to make.

MAKES 4 PORTIONS

1 sweet potato (about 6 oz), peeled and cut into chunks

a good pinch of powdered cinnamon
a few tablespoons baby milk

Cover the sweet-potato chunks with water, bring to a boil, and simmer for about 30 minutes or until soft. Drain and mash together with the cinnamon and enough baby milk to make the desired consistency.

Leek, Sweet Potato, and Pea Purée

Sweet potatoes make perfect baby food; they are full of nutrients and have a naturally sweet taste and smooth texture. Choose the orange-fleshed variety as it is rich in beta-carotene. It is fine to use frozen vegetables in baby purées as they are frozen within hours of being picked and can be just as nutritious as fresh vegetables. Once cooked, frozen vegetables can be refrozen.

MAKES 5 PORTIONS

³/₄ cup leek, washed and sliced
3¹/₂ cups sweet potato, peeled and chopped

1¹/₄ cups vegetable broth
¹/₂ cup frozen peas

Put the leek and sweet potato in a saucepan, pour over the vegetable broth, and bring to a boil. Cover and simmer for 15 minutes. Add the peas and continue to cook for 5 minutes. Purée in a blender.

FIRST TASTES MEAL PLANNER

Week 1	Early morning	Breakfast	Lunch	Dinner	Bedtime
Days 1–2	Breast/bottle	Breast/bottle	Breast/bottle Baby rice	Breast/bottle	Breast/bottle
Days 3–4	Breast/bottle	Breast/bottle	Breast/bottle Root vegetable e.g. carrot or sweet potato	Breast/bottle	Breast/bottle
Day 5	Breast/bottle	Breast/bottle	Breast/bottle Pear with baby rice	Breast/bottle	Breast/bottle
Day 6	Breast/bottle	Breast/bottle	Breast/bottle Apple	Breast/bottle	Breast/bottle
Day 7	Breast/bottle	Breast/bottle	Breast/bottle Vegetable e.g. butternut squash or sweet potato	Breast/bottle	Breast/bottle
Week 2					
Days 1–2	Breast/bottle Apple or pear with baby rice	Breast/bottle	Breast/bottle Root vegetable e.g. potato, parsnip or carrot	Breast/bottle	Breast/bottle
Days 3–4	Breast/bottle Banana or papaya	Breast/bottle	Breast/bottle **Sweet Vegetable Medley**	Breast/bottle	Breast/bottle
Days 5–6	Breast/bottle Apple or pear	Breast/bottle	Breast/bottle Sweet potato, butternut squash or rutabaga	Breast/bottle	Breast/bottle
Day 7	Breast/bottle Peach and banana or mashed banana	Breast/bottle	Breast/bottle Carrot or carrot and parsnip	Breast/bottle	Breast/bottle

These charts are intended only as a guide and will depend on many factors including weight. Some babies may only want one solid feed a day and some may prefer to have a second meal at supper time. Bold type indicates recipes shown in the book.

FIRST TASTES MEAL PLANNER

Week 3	Early morning	Breakfast	Lunch	Dinner	Bedtime
Day 1	Breast/bottle	Breast/bottle Banana	Diluted juice or water **Sweet Vegetable Medley**	Breast/bottle	Breast/bottle
Day 2	Breast/bottle	Breast/bottle Apple	Diluted juice or water **Sweet Vegetable Medley**	Breast/bottle	Breast/bottle
Day 3	Breast/bottle	Breast/bottle **Peaches, Apples, and Pears**	Diluted juice or water **Broccoli Trio**	Breast/bottle	Breast/bottle
Day 4	Breast/bottle	Breast/bottle **Cream of Fruit**	Diluted juice or water **Butternut Squash and Pear**	Breast/bottle	Breast/bottle
Day 5	Breast/bottle	Breast/bottle **Cream of Fruit**	Diluted juice or water **Butternut Squash and Pear**	Breast/bottle	Breast/bottle
Day 6	Breast/bottle	Breast/bottle Banana or papaya	Diluted juice or water **Potato, Zucchini, and Broccoli**	Breast/bottle	Breast/bottle
Day 7	Breast/bottle	Breast/bottle Pear or baby rice	Diluted juice or water **Carrot and Pea Purée**	Breast/bottle	Breast/bottle

Fruit juice should be diluted at least three parts water to one part juice, or substituted completely, with cooled, boiled water.

AFTER FIRST TASTES ACCEPTED MEAL PLANNER

	Early morning	*Breakfast*	*Lunch*	*Dinner*	*Bedtime*
Day 1	Breast/bottle	Breast/bottle **Three-Fruit Purée**	**Leek, Sweet Potato, and Pea Purée** Breast/bottle	**Carrot and Cauliflower** Water or diluted juice	Breast/bottle
Day 2	Breast/bottle	Breast/bottle **Three-Fruit Purée**	**Leek, Sweet Potato, and Pea Purée** Breast/bottle	**Sweet Vegetable Medley** Water or diluted juice	Breast/bottle
Day 3	Breast/bottle	Breast/bottle Pear and baby cereal	**Broccoli Trio** Breast/bottle	Sweet potato Water or diluted juice	Breast/bottle
Day 4	Breast/bottle	Breast/bottle **Apple and Cinnamon**	**Baby Cereal and Vegetables** Breast/bottle	Sweet potato Water or diluted juice	Breast/bottle
Day 5	Breast/bottle	Breast/bottle **Apple and Cinnamon** and baby cereal	**Avocado and Banana** Breast/bottle	**Carrot and Pea Purée** Water or diluted juice	Breast/bottle
Day 6	Breast/bottle	Breast/bottle Banana	**Watercress, Potato, and Zucchini Purée** Breast/bottle	**Broccoli Trio** Water or diluted juice	Breast/bottle
Day 7	Breast/bottle	Breast/bottle **Apple and Banana with Orange Juice**	**Watercress, Potato, and Zucchini Purée** Breast/bottle	**Broccoli Trio** Water or diluted juice	Breast/bottle

These charts are intended only as a guide and will depend on many factors including weight. Some babies will manage to eat some fruit after lunch and dinner.

AFTER FIRST TASTES ACCEPTED MEAL PLANNER

	Breakfast	*Mid-morning*	*Lunch*	*Mid-afternoon*	*Dinner*	*Bedtime*
Day 1	Breast/bottle Baby cereal Mashed banana	Breast/bottle	**Leek, Sweet Potato, and Pea Purée** Water or diluted juice	Breast/bottle	Carrot Pear or peach Teething biscuit Water or diluted juice	Breast/bottle
Day 2	Breast/bottle Baby cereal **Apple and Raisin Compote**	Breast/bottle	**Avocado and Banana** Water or diluted juice	Breast/bottle	**Carrot and Pea Purée** Finely chopped melon or plum Water or diluted juice	Breast/bottle
Day 3	Breast/bottle Baby cereal **Apple and Banana with Orange Juice**	Breast/bottle	**Sweet Potato with Cinnamon** Water or diluted juice	Breast/bottle	**Potato, Zucchini, and Broccoli** **Mixed Dried-Fruit Compote** Water or diluted juice	Breast/bottle
Day 4	Breast/bottle Baby cereal Yogurt	Breast/bottle	**Broccoli Trio** Water or diluted juice	Breast/bottle	**Sweet Vegetable Medley** Mango or papaya Water or diluted juice	Breast/bottle
Day 5	Breast/bottle Baby cereal **Peaches, Apples, and Pears**	Breast/bottle	**Broccoli Trio** Water or diluted juice	Breast/bottle	**Sweet Vegetable Medley** Fingers of toast Yogurt Water or diluted juice	Breast/bottle
Day 6	Breast/bottle Baby cereal **Peaches, Apples, and Pears**	Breast/bottle	**Watercress, Potato, and Zucchini Purée** Water or diluted juice	Breast/bottle	**Leek, Sweet Potato, and Pea Purée** Banana Water or diluted juice	Breast/bottle
Day 7	Breast/bottle Baby cereal **Apricot and Pear**	Breast/bottle	**Carrot and Pea Purée** Water or diluted juice	Breast/bottle	**Watercress, Potato, and Zucchini Purée** Peach and Banana Water or diluted juice	Breast/bottle

Fruit juice should be diluted at least three parts water to one part juice, or substituted completely, with cooled, boiled water.

CHAPTER THREE

SECOND-STAGE WEANING

Between six and nine months is a rapid development period for your baby. A six-month-old baby still needs to be supported while you are feeding him and, more often than not, still has no teeth. A nine-month-old baby, however, is usually strong enough to sit in a high chair while he is being fed and has already cut a few teeth. Babies of eight months are usually quite good at holding food themselves and enjoy eating small finger foods such as pieces of raw or cooked vegetables, pasta, or raw fruits. (Turn to pages 75–78 for suitable finger foods for young babies.) Babies are born with a store of iron that lasts for about six months. After this, they rely on their diet for the iron they need. If a baby doesn't have at least 18 fl oz (2¼ cups) breast milk or infant formula per day, his daily intake of iron is likely to be below the recommended level, and this can impair his mental and physical development. It is particularly important not to use ordinary cow's milk for your baby's regular drink before the age of one year as it doesn't contain as much iron or vitamins as formula milk.

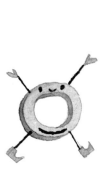
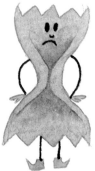
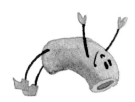

LESS MILK, MORE APPETITE

Once your baby is seven to eight months old, you can start cutting down on his milk feeds so that he is more hungry for his solids. However, between six months and one year, babies should have 16–25 fl oz (2–3 cups) breast milk or infant formula per day. In addition, you can give other dairy products, and offer water, diluted fruit juice or low-sugar herbal drinks with meals if your baby seems thirsty.

It is best to only put formula, breast milk, or water into your baby's bottle. Comfort-sucking on sweetened drinks is the main cause of tooth decay in young children, and babies are more vulnerable to decay than children or adults. You should start using a lidded cup with a soft spout and easy-to-hold handles once your baby is six months old. There are training cups available to guide your baby from a soft spout to open drinking cup in easy stages.

Let your baby's appetite determine how much he eats and never force him to eat something he actually dislikes. Do not offer it for a while, but reintroduce it a few weeks later. You may find that second time around he loves it.

Remember that at this age it is normal for babies to be quite chubby. As soon as your baby starts crawling and walking, he will lose this excess weight.

THE FOODS TO CHOOSE

Your baby can now eat protein foods like eggs, cheese, legumes, chicken, and fish.

Limit any foods that might be indigestible, such as spinach, lentils, cheese, berries, or citrus fruits, and do not worry if some foods, like legumes, peas, and raisins, pass through your child undigested; until they are about two years old, babies cannot completely digest husked vegetables and the skins of fruits. Of course, peeling, mashing, and puréeing fruit and vegetables will aid digestion. With foods like bread, flour, pasta, and rice, try to choose whole-grain (rather than refined) as it is more nutritious.

Once your baby has passed the six-month stage and is happily eating slightly coarser-textured foods, there is no need to continue giving him special baby cereals. You can use adult cereals, such as instant oatmeal, Grahams, and Chex, which are just as nutritious and much cheaper. Choose a cereal that isn't highly refined and is low in sugar and salt. Many people use commercial baby foods because they are easy to prepare; they also think, due to the long list of vitamins and minerals on the box, that they are more nutritious. However, babies who eat a well-balanced diet of fresh foods get a perfectly adequate quantity of vitamins and minerals. Also, baby foods in general are heavily processed, and their finer texture and bland flavors hinder the development of your baby's tastes.

Beware, too, of some of the teething biscuits you can buy, which are supposedly the "ideal food for your baby." They are full of sugar (often the amount isn't even stated on the list of ingredients). Give your baby some toast to chew on or follow the recipe for teething biscuits in the nine-to-twelve-months finger-food section (see page 76).

Ordinary cow's milk isn't suitable as your baby's main drink for the first year, as it doesn't contain enough nutrients for proper growth. However, whole cow's milk can be used in cooking or with cereal.

Fruit

Your baby should now be able to eat all fruits, and both fresh and dried fruits make a great snack. Different fruits contain different vitamins, so include as much variety as possible. Dried fruits are also a good source of other nutrients and energy. Take care to remove any pits before giving fruit, and don't give whole grapes to young babies as they may choke on them.

Vitamin C boosts iron absorption so it's important to include vitamin C-rich fruits like citrus or berry fruits in your child's diet. It's good to give cereal with diluted orange juice in the morning. It also combines well with savory foods like carrot, fish, and liver.

To begin with, give berry and citrus fruits in small quantities as they can be indigestible, and babies can have an adverse reaction to them. Combine them with other fruits like apple, banana, pear, or peach. Kiwi fruit can also cause an allergic reaction in some young children. This is rare, but do watch your baby closely, especially if there is a family history of allergies or conditions such as eczema or asthma.

Vegetables

Your baby is now able to eat all vegetables, but if certain flavors – like that of spinach or broccoli – are too strong, try mixing them together with a cheese sauce or with root vegetables like sweet potato, carrot, or potato. Combinations of vegetables and fruit are also good – try butternut squash and apple, or spinach and pear. Steamed vegetables, like carrot sticks or small florets of cauliflower, make good finger food.

Frozen vegetables reach the freezer within hours of being picked, and often retain as many nutrients as fresh ones. They are fine for making baby food and, once cooked, can be refrozen.

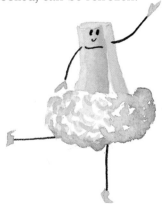

Eggs

Eggs are an excellent source of protein and also contain iron and zinc. They can be given from six months, but don't serve raw or lightly cooked eggs to babies under one year as there is a risk of salmonella.

The white and yolk should be cooked until solid. Hard-boiled eggs, omelets, and well-cooked scrambled eggs are quick to cook and nutritious.

Fish

Many children grow up disliking fish, as they find it bland and boring. Counteract this by mixing it with stronger tastes, such as cheese or herbs. If your child gets excited at the prospect of fish for supper, then you deserve to be a very proud parent indeed.

Oily fish like salmon, mackerel, fresh tuna, and sardines is particularly important for brain and visual development. Ideally, these should be included in the diet twice a week.

If fish is overcooked, it becomes tough and tasteless. It is cooked when it just flakes with a fork but is still firm. Always check very carefully for bones before serving.

Meat

Chicken is an ideal first meat. It blends well with root vegetables like carrot and sweet potato, which give chicken purée a smooth texture. Chicken also works well with fruits like apple and grape. Homemade chicken broth forms the basis of many recipes so I recommend that you make large batches. It will keep in the refrigerator for 3–4 days.

Iron is important for brain development; babies require the most iron between six months and two years. Iron-deficiency anaemia is the most common nutritional problem during early childhood, but the symptoms can be hard to detect. Your baby may just be tired and pale and more prone to infection, or his growth and development may seem to slow down. Red meat provides the best source of iron, in particular liver, which is ideal for babies as it has a soft texture and is easy to digest. Babies often reject red meats because of the chewy texture. Try combining it with root vegetables or pasta, as they help to produce a texture that is much smoother and easier to swallow.

Pasta

Pasta tends to be a favorite with babies and young children. It's a good source of carbohydrate, and adding tiny pasta shapes to purées when your baby is about eight months is a good way to encourage chewing. Many vegetable purées make good pasta sauces, to which you could add a little grated cheese. Either buy tiny pasta shapes or chop up spaghetti. Also try couscous, which has a soft texture perfect for babies. It is quick to cook and combines well with diced chicken or vegetables.

TEXTURES

You shouldn't give smooth purées to your baby for too long as it is important that he learns to chew. As teeth begin to emerge, give coarser purées and grated, mashed, and finely chopped food. Initially, babies often refuse to eat food that has lumps in it. If this happens, try adding pasta to purées as mentioned above, or give tender steamed vegetables or fruit as finger food.

FRUIT

Going Bananas

Babies love bananas and this recipe is scrumptious. Delicious served with vanilla ice cream.

MAKES 1 PORTION

1 teaspoon butter
1 small banana, peeled and sliced

a pinch of powdered cinnamon
2 tablespoons fresh orange juice

Melt the butter in a small skillet. Stir in the sliced banana, sprinkle with a little cinnamon and sauté for 2 minutes. Pour in the orange juice and continue cooking for 2 minutes. Mash with a fork.

Banana and Blueberry

Bananas combine well with lots of different fruits. Try, also, peach, mango, dried apricot, or prune. You can also mix banana and fruit combinations with some full-fat plain yogurt. Serve straight away, before the banana turns brown.

MAKES 1 PORTION

¼ cup blueberries
1 tablespoon water

1 small, ripe banana, peeled and sliced

Put the blueberries into a saucepan with the water and cook for about 2 minutes or until the fruit just starts to burst open. Whizz with a hand blender, together with the sliced banana, until smooth.

Peach, Apple, and Strawberry Purée

You could also make Apple, Strawberry, and Blueberry Purée using $^1/_4$ cup blueberries instead of peach.

MAKES 2 PORTIONS

1 large apple, peeled, cored, and chopped
1 large ripe peach, peeled, pitted,
and chopped

$^3/_4$ cup strawberries, halved
1 tablespoon baby rice

Steam the apple for about 4 minutes. Add the peach and strawberries to the steamer and continue to cook for about 3 minutes. Blend the fruits to a smooth purée and stir in the baby rice.

Peaches and Rice

You could also combine the cooked rice with other fruits like dried apricots (chop and simmer with the rice), or plums cooked with a little sugar.

MAKES 2 PORTIONS

1 tablespoon flaked brown rice
$^5/_8$ cup milk
1 ripe peach, skinned, pitted, and chopped

Put the rice and milk in a small pan. Stir over a low heat for about 5 minutes or until it boils and thickens. Simmer for 5 minutes, then stir in the chopped peach. Purée for young babies.

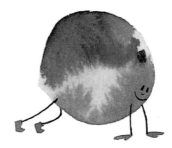

Apricot, Apple, and Peach Purée

Dried apricots are a concentrated form of nutrients. They are rich in iron, potassium, and beta-carotene, and babies tend to like their sweet flavor.

MAKES 5 PORTIONS

⅔ cup ready-to-eat dried apricots
2 dessert apples, peeled, cored,
and chopped

1 large, ripe peach, skinned, pitted, and
chopped, or 1 ripe pear, peeled, cored,
and chopped

Put the apricots into a small saucepan and cover with water. Cook over a gentle heat for 5 minutes. Add the chopped apples and continue to cook for 5 minutes. Purée together with the peach or pear.

Yogurt and Fruit

It's important to make sure that as well as fruit and vegetables, your baby gets enough fat in his diet. Recipes like vegetables in cheese sauce and fruit mixes with Greek yogurt are very good for your baby.

MAKES 1 PORTION

fresh fruit, e.g. 1 ripe peach, small mango,
or a combination like mango and banana

2 tablespoons full-fat plain yogurt
a little maple syrup (optional)

Peel the fruit, remove any pits, mash the flesh, and mix with the yogurt. Stir in a little maple syrup to sweeten if necessary.

Homemade Fruit Gelatin

It's easy to make gelatin with delicious fruit juices and fresh fruit. Personally, I prefer to use 4 sheets of leaf gelatin rather than gelatin powder (see method below), so I would recommend you try this.

MAKES 4 PORTIONS

2½ cups cranberry and raspberry juice
1 sachet powdered gelatin

2 tablespoons superfine sugar
1 cup fresh raspberries

Place half of the juice in a small saucepan and heat until just at boiling point. Remove from the heat and stir in the powdered gelatin and superfine sugar until dissolved. If not completely dissolved, stir over a low heat but do not boil. Pour this into the remaining cold juice and then pour into a serving dish and stir in the raspberries. Refrigerate until set.

Blood Orange Gelatin

Leaf gelatin dissolves like a dream and is fantastic for making gelatin.

MAKES 4 PORTIONS

4 leaves gelatin
2½ cups freshly squeezed

blood-orange juice
3 tablespoons superfine sugar

Break the gelatin leaves into a shallow dish (use 6 leaves if using a mold). Pour over 6 tablespoons juice. Heat the remaining juice until very hot but not boiling, and stir in the sugar until dissolved. Remove from the heat. Little by little, remove the softened gelatin leaves from the dish and stir into the hot juice. The leaves will disappear. Stir in any juice left in the dish. Leave to cool. Pour the juice into a bowl, individual glasses, or gelatin mold. Chill until set.

VEGETABLES

Lovely Lentils

Lentils are a good cheap source of protein. They also provide iron, which is very important for brain development, particularly between the ages of six months and two years. Lentils can be difficult for young babies to digest and should be combined with plenty of fresh vegetables as in this recipe. This tasty purée also makes a delicious soup for the family by simply adding more broth and some seasoning.

MAKES 8 PORTIONS

¼ small onion, finely chopped
1 cup carrot, chopped
¼ cup celery, chopped
1 tablespoon vegetable oil

¼ cup split red lentils
1¾ cups sweet potato, peeled and chopped
1¾ cups vegetable or chicken broth
(see page 33 or 62) or water

Sauté the onion, carrot, and celery in the vegetable oil for about 5 minutes or until softened. Add the lentils and sweet potato and pour over the broth or water. Bring to a boil, turn down the heat, and simmer, covered, for 20 minutes. Purée in a blender.

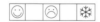

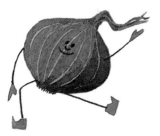

Tomatoes and Carrots with Basil

If you introduce your baby to new flavors at an early age, he will tend to grow up a less fussy eater.

MAKES 4 PORTIONS

1¼ cups carrot, peeled and sliced
1 cup cauliflower, cut into florets
1½ tablespoons butter

7 oz ripe tomatoes, skinned, seeded, and roughly chopped
2–3 fresh basil leaves
½ cup Cheddar cheese, grated

Put the carrot in a small saucepan, cover with boiling water, and simmer, covered, for 10 minutes. Add the cauliflower and cook, covered, for 7–8 minutes, adding extra water if necessary. Meanwhile, melt the butter, add the tomatoes and sauté until mushy. Stir in the basil and cheese until melted. Purée the carrot and cauliflower with about 3 tablespoons of the cooking liquid and the tomato sauce.

Baked Sweet Potato with Orange

Sweet potatoes are delicious baked either in the oven or microwave and then combined with fruit, such as apple or peach purée. They are a good source of carbohydrate, vitamins, and minerals.

MAKES 8 PORTIONS

1 medium sweet potato, scrubbed
2 tablespoons fresh orange juice

2 tablespoons milk

Cook the sweet potato on a cookie sheet in an oven preheated to 400°F for about 1 hour or until tender. Cool a little, then scoop out the flesh. Purée or mash with the orange juice and milk until smooth.

Sweet Potato with Spinach and Peas

This purée makes a tasty introduction to spinach for your baby.

MAKES 5 PORTIONS

1¼ tablespoons butter
¾ cup leek, finely sliced
1 sweet potato (about 13 oz), peeled
and chopped

⅞ cup water
½ cup frozen peas
½ cup fresh baby spinach, washed and
any tough stalks removed

Melt the butter in a saucepan and sauté the leek for 2–3 minutes or until softened. Add the sweet potato. Pour over the water, bring to a boil, then cover and simmer for 7–8 minutes. Add the peas and spinach and cook for 3 minutes. Purée the vegetables in a blender to make a smooth consistency for your baby.

Sweet Vegetable Purée

Although vegetables like corn and peas have a sweet taste that babies like, they should be puréed in a food mill as the husks are indigestible.

MAKES 3 PORTIONS

¼ cup onion, chopped
¾ cup carrot, peeled and chopped
1 tablespoon olive oil
1¼ cups potato, peeled and chopped

⅞ cup water
2 tablespoons frozen corn kernels
1 tablespoon frozen peas

Fry the onion and carrot gently in the oil for 5 minutes. Stir in the potato, add the water, bring to a boil, then cover and simmer for 10 minutes. Add the corn and peas and simmer for about 5 minutes. Purée in a food mill.

Trio of Cauliflower, Red Bell Pepper, and Corn

Babies like the bright colors and natural sweetness of these vegetables. Always purée corn in a mill for young babies to get rid of the tough outer skin.

MAKES 4 PORTIONS

1 cup cauliflower, broken into small florets
½ cup milk

½ cup Cheddar cheese, grated
½ cup red bell pepper, chopped
½ cup frozen corn kernels

Put the cauliflower in a small saucepan with the milk and cook over a low heat for about 8 minutes until tender. Stir in the grated cheese until melted. Meanwhile, steam the bell pepper and corn or cook in some water in a small saucepan for about 6 minutes until tender. Drain the corn and bell pepper. Purée together with the cauliflower, milk, and cheese in a food mill.

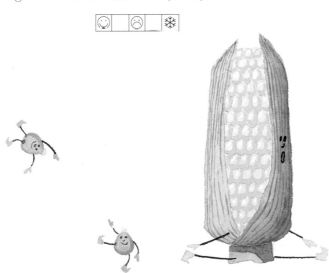

Cauliflower Cheese

This is a great favorite with babies. Try using different cheeses or combinations of cheese until you find your baby's favorite taste. The cheese sauce can be used over a mixture of vegetables as well.

MAKES 5 PORTIONS

1¹/₂ cups cauliflower florets

Cheese Sauce
1 tablespoon margarine
1 tablespoon cornstarch
⁵/₈ cup milk
¹/₂ cup grated Cheddar, Edam, or Swiss cheese

Wash the cauliflower florets carefully and steam until tender (about 10 minutes). Meanwhile, for the sauce, melt the margarine over a gentle heat in a heavy-bottomed saucepan and stir in the cornstarch to make a smooth paste. Add the milk and stir until thickened. Take the saucepan off the heat and stir in the grated cheese. Keep stirring until all the cheese has melted and the sauce is smooth.

Add the cauliflower to the sauce and purée in a blender for younger babies. For older babies, mash with a fork or chop into little pieces.

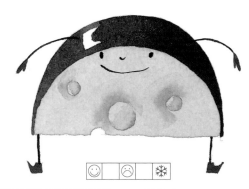

Zucchini Gratin

This creamy purée is also good using green beans or broccoli.

MAKES 6 PORTIONS

*1 medium potato (about 4 oz), peeled
and chopped*
1¹/₂ cups zucchini, sliced

a little butter
³/₈ cup Cheddar or Swiss cheese, grated
4 tablespoons milk

Boil the potato until soft. Steam the zucchini for 8 minutes. Drain the potato, add the butter and cheese, and stir until melted. Purée the potato mixture, zucchini, and milk with an electric hand blender.

Leek and Potato Purée

This was Lara's favorite vegetable purée. It also makes a delicious soup for adults if you add seasoning.

MAKES 4 PORTIONS

2 tablespoons butter
1⁵/₈ cups leek, finely sliced
2¹/₄ cups potato, peeled and chopped

1¹/₄ cups chicken broth (see page 62)
2 tablespoons Greek yogurt

Heat the margarine or oil in a heavy-based pan. Add the leek and cook over a gentle heat for 10 minutes until softened, stirring occasionally. Add the diced potato and broth and simmer, covered, for 25–30 minutes until tender. Purée, and stir in the Greek yogurt.

Zucchini and Pea Soup

When I experimented with this combination, the baby purée turned out to be so good that I also made a delicious soup for the rest of the family. Simply increase the quantities and add extra broth and seasoning.

MAKES 4 PORTIONS

½ onion, peeled and finely chopped
1 tablespoon butter or margarine
½ cup zucchini, trimmed and thinly sliced

1 medium potato (about 5 oz), peeled and chopped
½ cup chicken or vegetable broth (see page 62)
¼ cup frozen peas

Sauté the onion in the butter or margarine until softened. Add the zucchini, potato, and broth. Bring to a boil, then cover and simmer gently for 12 minutes. Add the frozen peas, bring to a boil, then reduce the heat and continue to cook for 5 minutes. Purée in a blender.

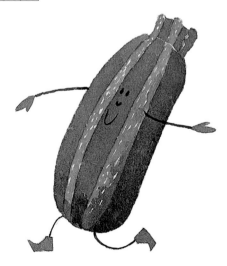

Minestrone

The vegetables in minestrone soup add texture but are nice and soft for your baby to chew. However, for younger babies you could blend this soup to the desired texture. Add a little seasoning and some extra broth to make this into a delicious soup for the rest of the family.

MAKES 4 ADULT PORTIONS OR 12 BABY PORTIONS

1 tablespoon vegetable oil
½ small onion, peeled and finely chopped
½ leek, white part only, washed and finely chopped
1 medium carrot, peeled and diced
½ celery stalk, diced
1 cup green beans, cut into ½-inch lengths

1 potato, peeled and diced
1 tablespoon fresh parsley, finely chopped
2 teaspoons tomato paste
5 cups chicken or vegetable broth (see pages 62 and 33)
3 tablespoons frozen peas
⅓ cup very small pasta shapes

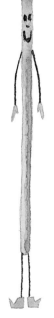

Heat the oil in a saucepan and fry the onion and leek for 2 minutes, then add the carrot, celery, green beans, potato, and parsley and sauté for 4 minutes. Stir in the tomato paste and cook for 1 minute. Pour over the chicken or vegetable broth and simmer, covered, for 20 minutes. Add the frozen peas and pasta and cook for 5 minutes (check the packet instructions for the cooking time of the pasta).

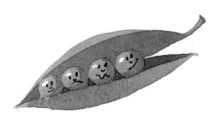

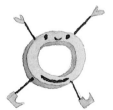

FISH

Flounder with Tomatoes and Potato

This makes a good, creamy-textured fish purée.

MAKES 4 PORTIONS

1 flounder, filleted and skinned
2 medium tomatoes, skinned, seeded,
and chopped
a little margarine or butter

1 bay leaf
½ cup milk
1 small potato, peeled

Put the flounder into a dish, cover with the tomatoes, dot with the margarine or butter, and add the bay leaf. Pour over most of the milk. Cover with foil and cook in an oven preheated to 350°F for 20 minutes. (Alternately, cover with a lid and cook in the microwave on High for about 3 minutes.)

While the fish is cooking, boil the potato. When soft, mash it with the remaining milk and margarine or butter. Flake the fish when it is cooked, remove the bay leaf, and mash or purée the fish together with the liquid in which it was cooked. You can either mix in the mashed potato or serve it as an accompaniment to the fish.

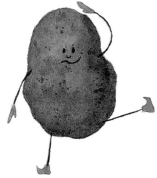

Flounder in Cheese Sauce

Fish and cheese sauce go really well together, and the combination is always popular. Add some chives and you give an old recipe a new taste.

MAKES 6 PORTIONS

6 oz flounder, filleted and skinned
3 tablespoons milk
1 bay leaf
a little butter

Cheese Sauce
2 tablespoons butter
2 tablespoons all-purpose flour
¾ cup milk
¾ cup Cheddar cheese, grated
1 teaspoon snipped chives or
chopped parsley

Put the flounder fillets in a suitable dish with the milk and bay leaf and dot with butter. Cover and microwave on High for about 4 minutes. Alternately, poach the fish in milk, in a saucepan, until cooked.

To prepare the sauce, melt the butter and stir in the flour. Cook for 1 minute, then gradually whisk in the milk, cooking over a gentle heat until you have a smooth white sauce. Bring to a boil and simmer for 1 minute, stirring constantly. Remove from the heat and stir in the cheese until melted. Add the snipped chives or parsley.

Flake the fish with a fork and make sure there are no stray bones. Add the fish to the cheese sauce and put it through the food mill, or mash, or purée in a blender.

Flounder with Spinach and Cheese

Frozen vegetables are a good alternative to fresh, and can often be more nutritious than ones that have been kept in the kitchen for several days.

MAKES 8 PORTIONS

8 oz flounder, filleted and skinned
1 tablespoon milk
1 bay leaf
a few peppercorns
a little butter
1 cup fresh spinach, or ¹/₂ cup frozen

Cheese Sauce
2 tablespoons butter
2 tablespoons all-purpose flour
³/₄ cup milk
¹/₂ cup Swiss cheese, grated

Put the flounder in a suitable dish with the milk, bay leaf, peppercorns, and butter. Microwave for about 3 minutes on High, or poach in a saucepan for 3–4 minutes with the milk for the sauce (strain the milk afterwards, ready to make the sauce). Meanwhile, cook the spinach in a saucepan with just a little water for about 3 minutes, or cook frozen spinach according to the box directions. Squeeze out the excess water. Make the cheese sauce (see page 59). Discard the bay leaf and peppercorns, flake the fish carefully, and purée with the spinach and cheese sauce.

Fillet of Cod with Sweet Potato

The orange-fleshed sweet potato is an excellent source of beta-carotene, which may help to prevent certain types of cancer. Babies tend to love the taste of sweet potato, so this recipe makes a good introduction to fish.

MAKES 8 PORTIONS

2 cups sweet potato, peeled
3 oz cod, filleted and skinned
2 tablespoons milk

a little butter
juice of 1 orange (about ¹/₂ cup)

Put the sweet potato in a saucepan, just cover with water, bring to a boil, then cover and simmer for 20 minutes until soft. Put the fish in a suitable dish, add the milk, dot with butter, cover and microwave on High for 2 minutes until the fish is cooked. Alternately, poach in a saucepan with the milk and butter for 6–7 minutes. Put the cooked sweet potato, drained fish, and orange juice into a blender and purée until smooth.

Fillet of Fish in an Orange Sauce

This is one of my family's favorite fish recipes. Do not be put off by the odd combination, as it gives a marvellous rich taste.

MAKES 5 PORTIONS

8 oz white fish, filleted and skinned
juice of 1 orange (about ½ cup)
½ cup Cheddar cheese, grated

2 teaspoons fresh parsley, finely chopped
1 cup cornflakes, crushed
a little margarine

Put the fish in a greased dish, cover with the orange juice, cheese, parsley, and cornflakes, and dot with the margarine. Cover with foil and bake in an oven preheated to 350°F for about 20 minutes. Alternately, cover with a lid and cook in a microwave on High for 4 minutes.

Flake the fish carefully, checking for any bones, and mash everything together with the liquid in which the fish was cooked.

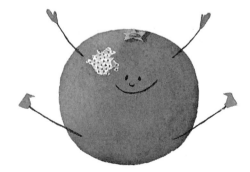

CHICKEN

Chicken Broth and My First Chicken Purée

Bouillon cubes are unsuitable for babies under a year as they are high in salt, so I make my own chicken broth and use it as a base for chicken and vegetable purées. It keeps in the refrigerator for 3 days. For babies over one year you can add 3 chicken bouillon cubes for a stronger flavor. Instead of a boiling fowl, you could use the carcass from a roast chicken.

MAKES APPROXIMATELY 4 PINTS

1 large boiling fowl, plus giblets
4 pints water
2 parsnips
3 large carrots
2 leeks

2 large onions
1 celery stalk
2 sprigs of fresh parsley
1 sachet bouquet garni

Cut the chicken into 8 pieces, trimming any excess fat. Trim, peel, and wash the vegetables as necessary. Put the chicken pieces into a large saucepan together with the giblets. Cover with 4 pints water, bring to a boil, and skim the froth from the top. Add the vegetables and parsley and simmer for about 3 hours. It is best to remove the chicken breasts after about 1½ hours if you are going to eat them; otherwise they will become too dry. Leave in the refrigerator overnight and remove any congealed fat from the top in the morning. Strain the chicken and vegetables to make the chicken broth. Season to taste.

You can purée some of the chicken breast in a mill together with a selection of the vegetables and some broth to make a chicken and vegetable purée. This also makes a wonderful clear chicken soup (with added bouillon cubes and seasoning) for older babies and you can add some thin noodles.

Chicken with Cottage Cheese

Babies of this age are a little too young to eat pieces of chicken as finger food. This and the following four recipes show you simple ways of transforming cold chicken into tasty food for your baby.

MAKES 2 PORTIONS

2 oz cooked boneless chicken, chopped
1 tablespoon plain yogurt

1½ tablespoons cottage cheese with pineapple

Mix together the chicken, yogurt, and cottage cheese. Put through a mill to make a smooth purée.

Chicken with Parsnip and Beans

If freezing this recipe, do not purée the chicken with the vegetables until they are cold. It is important to avoid warming the chicken.

MAKES 5 PORTIONS

½ cup parsnip, peeled and sliced
1 cup sweet potato, peeled and chopped
¼ cup green beans, topped and tailed

1½ oz boneless chicken, cooked
4 tablespoons chicken broth (see page 62) or milk

Put the vegetables into a saucepan, cover with water, bring to a boil, then cover and simmer until tender. Drain, then purée with the chicken and the broth or milk.

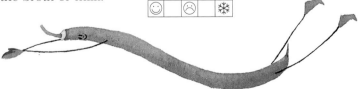

Chicken with Sweet Potato and Apple

This combination gives a smooth texture and sweet taste that babies like.

MAKES 4 PORTIONS

1 tablespoon butter
1/3 cup onion, chopped
4 oz chicken breast, chopped
1/2 dessert apple, peeled and chopped

1 sweet potato (about 11 oz), peeled and chopped
1 cup chicken broth (see page 62)

Melt the butter in a saucepan, add the onion, and sauté for 2–3 minutes. Add the chicken and sauté until it turns opaque. Add the apple, sweet potato, and broth. Bring to a boil, cover, and simmer for 15 minutes. Purée to the desired consistency.

☺ ☹ ❄

Chicken Salad Purée

What could be simpler? For toddlers, chop the ingredients, leave out the yogurt and mix with a little mayonnaise.

MAKES 1 PORTION

1 oz cooked boneless chicken
1 slice cucumber, peeled and chopped
1 small tomato, skinned, seeded, and chopped
2 oz avocado, peeled and chopped
4 seedless grapes, skinned
1 tablespoon plain yogurt

Put all the ingredients in a blender and purée to the desired consistency. Serve immediately.

☺ ☹

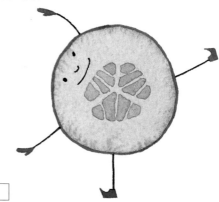

Chicken in Tomato Sauce

MAKES 12 PORTIONS

¼ cup onion, chopped
1 cup carrot, thinly sliced
1½ tablespoons vegetable oil
1 small chicken breast, cubed

1 cup potato, peeled and chopped
7 oz canned chopped tomatoes
½ cup chicken broth (see page 62)

Sauté the onion and carrot in the oil until softened, then add the chicken and potato and continue to cook for 3 minutes. Pour over the tomatoes together with the chicken broth. Bring to a boil, then cook over a gentle heat for about 30 minutes or until the potato is quite soft. Purée in a food mill or, for babies of nine months and older, chop in a blender. You could also add a little milk to make a smoother texture if you wish.

Easy One-Pot Chicken

This is an ideal purée for introducing young babies to chicken.

MAKES 12 PORTIONS

½ small onion, finely chopped
1 tablespoon butter
4 oz chicken breast, skinned, boned,
and cubed

1 medium carrot, trimmed and sliced
2½ cups sweet potato, peeled and chopped
1¼ cups chicken broth (see
page 62)

Sauté the onion in the butter until softened. Add the chicken and sauté for 3–4 minutes. Add the vegetables, pour over the broth, bring to a boil, and simmer, covered, for 30 minutes or until the chicken is cooked through and the vegetables are tender. Purée in a blender.

Chicken with Pumpkin and Grapes

Combining chicken with pumpkin and grapes gives it a little sweetness which babies love. This is very simple to make and is usually gobbled up pretty quickly.

MAKES 4 PORTIONS

1 tablespoon unsalted butter
1/2 cup leek, sliced
1 small chicken breast or 2 thighs,
skinned and off the bone

2 cups pumpkin, peeled and chopped
6 grapes, deseeded and peeled
3/4 cup chicken broth (see page 62)

Melt the butter in a saucepan and sauté the leek for 2 minutes. Cut the chicken into pieces and sauté with the leek for 3 minutes. Add the pumpkin and grapes, pour over the broth, and simmer, covered, for 15 minutes. Purée to the desired consistency using as much of the cooking liquid as necessary.

☺	☹	❄

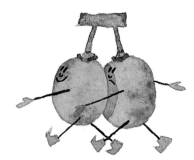

MEAT

Braised Beef with Sweet Potato

Both this and the recipe below make good introductions to red meat.

MAKES 6 PORTIONS

1 leek, washed and sliced
1¼ tablespoons butter
4 oz braising steak or lamb, cut into cubes
2 tablespoons flour

2½ cups sweet potato, peeled and chopped
1¼ cups chicken broth (see page 62)
juice of 1 orange (about ½ cup)

In a flameproof Dutch oven, soften the leek in the butter. Roll the meat in the flour and add to the leek to brown. Add the sweet potato, broth, and orange juice. Bring to a boil, cover, and transfer to an oven preheated to 350°F for 1¼ hours or until the meat is tender. Blend to the desired consistency.

Liver Special

MAKES 6 PORTIONS

3 oz calf's liver, or 2 chicken livers
½ cup chicken broth (see page 62)
½ cup leek, white part only, chopped
⅓ cup mushrooms, chopped

½ cup carrot, chopped
1 potato, peeled
a little butter
½ tablespoon milk

Trim and chop the liver and cook in the broth with the leek, mushrooms, and carrot for about 8 minutes over a low heat. Boil the potato until tender and mash with the butter and milk. Purée the liver and vegetables and mix with the potato.

PASTA

Tomato and Zucchini Pasta Stars

This tasty pasta sauce only takes about 10 minutes to prepare.

MAKES 3 PORTIONS

a scant ¼ cup pasta stars, uncooked
¾ cup zucchini, trimmed and diced
1½ tablespoons butter

3 medium tomatoes (about 7 oz),
skinned, seeded, and chopped
¼ cup Cheddar cheese, grated

Cook the pasta according to the packet instructions, or longer for young babies. Sauté the zucchini in the butter for about 5 minutes. Add the tomatoes and cook over a low heat for 5 minutes. Remove from the heat and stir in the cheese until melted. Purée in a blender and stir in the pasta.

Vegetable and Cheese Pasta Sauce

MAKES 3 PORTIONS OF SAUCE

⅝ cup carrot, peeled and sliced
⅜ cup broccoli florets
1½ tablespoons butter

2 tablespoons all-purpose flour
¾ cup milk
½ cup Cheddar cheese, grated

Steam the carrot for 10 minutes, then add the broccoli florets and cook for 7 minutes more. Meanwhile, melt the butter in a small saucepan and stir in the flour to make a thick paste. Gradually add the milk, bring to a boil and stir continuously until the sauce thickens. Simmer for 1 minute. Remove from the heat and stir in the grated cheese. Add the cooked vegetables to the cheese sauce and blend to a purée. Serve with tiny cooked pasta shapes.

My First Bolognese Sauce

A tasty recipe to encourage your baby to enjoy eating red meat.

MAKES 3 PORTIONS

1 tablespoon olive oil
1 small onion, peeled and chopped
1 garlic clove, crushed
1 large carrot (3½ oz), peeled
and grated
½ celery stalk, finely chopped

½ cup lean ground beef
⅔ cup mushrooms, chopped
3 medium tomatoes, skinned and chopped
½ tablespoon tomato paste
¾ cup unsalted chicken broth
3 tablespoons tiny pasta shapes

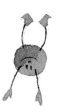

Heat the oil and sauté the onion, garlic, carrot, and celery for 5 minutes. Add the ground beef and sauté until browned, stirring occasionally. Add the mushrooms and sauté for 2 minutes. Stir in the tomatoes, tomato paste, and broth. Bring to a boil, then simmer for 15 minutes. Cook the pasta according to the box directions. Purée the sauce in a blender, drain the pasta, then mix with the sauce.

Tomato and Basil Pasta Sauce

Butterfly-shaped pasta is fun for babies to grasp in their hands.

MAKES 2 PORTIONS OF SAUCE

1 tablespoon butter
2 tablespoons onion, chopped
5 oz ripe tomatoes, skinned, seeded

and chopped
2 fresh basil leaves, torn
2 teaspoons cream cheese

Melt the butter in a saucepan and sauté the onion until softened. Add the tomatoes and sauté for 3 minutes or until mushy. Stir in the basil and cream cheese and heat through. Purée in a blender.

Napolitana Pasta Sauce

A tasty tomato sauce that goes well with all types of pasta – my children love this with ravioli stuffed with ricotta and spinach.

MAKES 4 PORTIONS OF SAUCE

1 tablespoon olive oil
½ small onion, peeled and chopped
½ garlic clove, peeled and crushed
½ cup carrot, peeled and chopped
1 cup passata

3 tablespoons water
2 fresh basil leaves, roughly torn
1 teaspoon Parmesan cheese, grated
1 teaspoon cream cheese

Heat the olive oil and sauté the onion, garlic, and carrot for 6 minutes. Add the passata, water, basil, and Parmesan. Cover and simmer for 15 minutes. Purée the sauce and stir in the cream cheese. Mix with pasta and serve.

Popeye Pasta

MAKES 4 PORTIONS

2 cups frozen or fresh spinach, washed and chopped
⅓ cup tiny pasta shapes (like soup pasta), uncooked

1 tablespoon butter
2 tablespoons milk
2 tablespoons cream cheese
½ cup Swiss cheese, grated

Cook the frozen spinach following box directions, or boil the fresh spinach in a little water for about 5 minutes. Press out the excess water. Cook the pasta according to the instructions on the box. Melt the butter and sauté the cooked spinach. Combine with the milk and cheeses, and chop finely in a food processor. Mix with the cooked pasta.

SECOND-STAGE WEANING MEAL PLANNER

	Breakfast	Mid-morning	Lunch	Mid-afternoon	Tea	Bedtime
Day 1	Chex with milk Mashed banana	Milk	**My First Chicken Purée** Grated apple Juice	Milk	**Leek and Potato Purée** Pear purée Water or juice	Milk
Day 2	Instant Oatmeal with milk Fruit purée Milk	Milk	**Flounder with Tomatoes and Potato** Mashed banana Juice	Milk	**Zucchini and Pea Soup** Yogurt Water or juice	Milk
Day 3	Apple purée and baby cereal Toast Milk	Milk	**Cauliflower Cheese** Grated pear Juice	Milk	**Braised Beef with Sweet Potato** Teething biscuit Water or juice	Milk
Day 4	Baby cereal with milk Dried apricot purée Yogurt	Milk	**Lovely Lentils** **Peaches and Rice** Juice	Milk	**Minestrone** Toast Water or juice	Milk
Day 5	Chex with milk **Peach, Apple, and Strawberry Purée**	Milk	Pasta with **Vegetable and Cheese Pasta Sauce** **Going Bananas** Juice	Milk	**My First Bolognese Sauce** Pear purée Water or juice	Milk
Day 6	Baby cereal with milk **Peach, Apple, and Strawberry Purée**	Milk	**Tomatoes and Carrots with Basil** **Homemade Fruit Gelatin** Juice	Milk	**Fillet of Fish in an Orange Sauce** Apple Water	Milk
Day 7	Oatmeal with milk **Yogurt and Fruit**	Milk	**Sweet Potato with Spinach and Peas** **Apricot, Apple, and Peach Purée** Juice	Milk	**Easy One-Pot Chicken** Papaya purée Water or juice	Milk

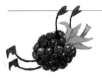

CHAPTER FOUR

NINE TO TWELVE MONTHS

Towards the end of the first year, a baby's weight gain usually slows down quite dramatically. Quite often, babies who have been good eaters in the past become much more difficult to feed. Many refuse to be spoon-fed and want to assert their new-found independence, using their hands to feed themselves. My older daughter at the age of ten months went through a phase of refusing to eat anything offered to her on a spoon. I was determined that she should eat the homemade purées I had prepared, so I gave her various finger foods, such as steamed carrots or strips of toast, which I dipped into the purées. That way I succeeded in getting her to eat and enjoy them, and everyone was happy.

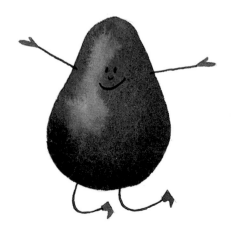

MEALTIME PATIENCE

Let your baby experiment by allowing her to use a spoon. Most of the food will probably end up on you or on the floor, but the more you allow your baby to experiment, the quicker she will master the art of feeding herself. Put a plastic splash mat under the high chair to catch the food that falls on the floor so that you can recycle it. It is probably best to have two bowls of food and two spoons: one that you use to spoon-feed your baby, the other (preferably a bowl which sticks to the table by suction) for your baby to play with.

You will need lots of patience at mealtimes, as many babies are very easily distracted at this stage and may prefer to play with their food rather than eat it. If all else fails, I find that if you can attract your baby's attention by giving her a small toy to hold, you can sometimes slip some food into her mouth on a spoon and then she will eat without really noticing what she is doing and will forget to put up any resistance!

No child under the age of one year needs to drink cow's milk. For drinks, continue using formula or breast milk, which has a much lower salt content and is complete with essential vitamins. However, as solid-food intake increases, milk need no longer form such a staple part of your child's diet, although she should still be drinking about 18 fl oz (2¼ cups) of milk a day (or the equivalent as dairy products or in cooking). It is an important source of protein and calcium. Many mothers assume that when their baby cries it is because she wants more milk but often babies of this age are given *too much* milk and not enough solid food. If you fill your baby's stomach with milk when she really wants some solid food, you will not get a very satisfied baby.

If you have a juice extractor, you can make all sorts of wonderful fruit and vegetable drinks for your baby – try combinations like apple, strawberry, and banana. Your baby should now be drinking happily from a cup. Keep the bottle for her bedtime drink of warm milk.

Your baby will be teething at this age and very often sore gums can put her off eating for a while. Don't worry, as she will make up for this later that day or the next day. (Rubbing a teething gel on your baby's gums, or giving her something very cold to chew, can help relieve soreness and restore appetite.)

It is a good idea to eat something with your baby at mealtimes. There are some mothers who sit opposite their babies and try to spoon food into their mouths while eating nothing themselves. Babies are great mimics and are more likely to enjoy eating if they see you tucking in as well.

THE FOODS TO CHOOSE

You can be a little more adventurous with the food that you make for your baby. It is a good idea now to develop her tastes for garlic and herbs, both of which are very healthful. Children tend to be less fussy eaters if they are introduced to a wide range of foods early. Again, if your baby dislikes certain foods, never force her to eat them; just leave out those foods and perhaps reintroduce them in a couple of days' time. Try also to vary the foods as much as possible, as this will lead to a more balanced diet. If you give your child a favorite food too often, it is possible she will go off it altogether.

Your baby can soon eat berry fruits (but these should still be put through a food mill in the earlier stages to get rid of the indigestible seeds). Fruit gelatins will be interesting for your baby to look at, feel, and eat. Your baby will like fruit and vegetables that have been grated.

Oily fish like salmon, sardines, and fresh tuna contains essential fatty acids and iron, so it is particularly good for your child. All fish must obviously be very fresh. Chicken dishes can become more interesting in both texture and taste, and the types of pasta cooked can be large enough for the independent baby to pick up (butterflies, spirals, shells, and animal shapes are good). Increase the quantity per serving of pasta to about $1/2$–$3/4$ cup cooked ($1/4$–$3/8$ cup dry).

Whenever possible, try to make the food look attractive on the plate. Choose contrasting colors and arrange the food in pretty shapes. You can use your imagination to make little faces or animals. Never pile too much food on to the plate but offer a second helping instead – your baby will let you know in no uncertain terms if she wants more.

Meat

Red meat is good for young children as it provides the best source of iron. If using ground meat, choose good-quality meat and ask your butcher to prepare it for you rather than buying it ready prepared. After cooking ground meat for young babies, I find that if I chop it in a food processor for 30 seconds, it becomes much softer and easier to chew. It's best not to give sausages or other processed meats, such as pâté or meat pies, to children.

TEXTURES AND QUANTITIES

It is easy to get into the habit of only giving your baby soft foods, but you should try to vary the consistency of the food that you offer. There is no need to purée all foods. Babies do not need teeth to be able to chew; gums do a great job on foods that are not too hard. Give some food mashed (fish), some grated (cheese), some diced (carrots), and some whole (pieces of chicken, slices of toast, and pieces of raw fruit).

As far as quantities are concerned, you must let your baby's appetite be your guide. You can start to freeze food in larger plastic containers and freeze individual portions like mini shepherd's pies in small ramekin dishes. Many meals that are included in this chapter can be enjoyed by the whole family, in which case adult-sized portions are given.

FINGER FOODS

By the age of nine months, your baby will probably want to start feeding herself. It is a good idea, therefore, to start giving her some foods that are easy for her to eat with her fingers. Finger foods are great for occupying your child while you prepare her meal – or you could make a whole meal of finger foods.

Never leave your child unattended while she is eating. It is very easy for a baby to choke on even very small pieces of food. Avoid giving your baby whole nuts, fruits that contain pits, whole grapes, ice cubes, olives, or any other foods that might get stuck in her throat.

What To Do If Your Baby Chokes

If your baby chokes, lay her face down on your forearm or lap with her head lower than her chest. Support her head and give her five light slaps between the shoulders with your free hand.

Raw Fruit

When giving your baby fruit, always make sure it has been peeled, and that any pits or seeds have been removed. If she finds it difficult to chew, give soft fruits that melt in the mouth such as banana, peach, or grated fruit. Berry and citrus fruit should only be given in small quantities to start with. Remove as much of the pith as possible.

Many babies who are teething enjoy biting into fruit. A banana put into the freezer for a few hours makes an excellent teething aid for young babies. Once your baby is able to hold food successfully, give her larger pieces of fruit and encourage her to bite off little bits. (But don't let her *store* these in her mouth; occasionally I had to resort to opening my son's mouth and removing food that he refused to swallow!) If your baby only has a few teeth, it is a good idea to give her grated fruit to chew.

FRUITY IDEAS

apple, apricot, avocado, banana, blueberries, cherries, grapes, kiwi fruit, mango, melon, nectarine, orange, papaya, peach, pear, plum, raspberries, strawberries, tomato

---

Dried Fruits

These are a good source of fiber, iron, and energy. Choose ready-to-eat fruits that are soft. Some dried apricots are treated with sulphur dioxide to preserve their bright-orange color; these should be avoided as they can trigger an asthma attack in susceptible babies. Don't give your baby lots of dried fruit as it can be difficult to digest – and laxative.

MORE FRUITY IDEAS

apple rings, apricots, banana chips, dates, peaches, pears, prunes, raisins, golden raisins

---

Vegetables

To begin with, give your baby soft, cooked vegetables cut into pieces that are easy for her to hold, and encourage her to bite off little pieces. (It is best to steam vegetables as this will help to preserve vitamin C.) Gradually cook the vegetables for less time so that your baby gets used to having to chew harder. Once your baby has good coordination, she will enjoy picking up little vegetables like peas and corn.

Once your baby has mastered the art of feeding herself cooked vegetables, you can introduce carefully washed, grated, raw vegetables and also sticks of raw vegetables. Even if your baby is unable to bite into these sticks, she will enjoy chewing on them as an aid to teething. Sticks of raw vegetables, such as carrots and cucumber, are very soothing for sore gums if they are chilled in the freezer or in iced water for a few minutes. Large pieces of raw vegetables are safer than small pieces as a baby will nibble off what she can manage, whereas a small piece put into her mouth whole could cause her to choke if she tried to swallow it.

When your baby can chew well, try giving her cooked corncobs. Cut the corn in half or into three pieces, or look out for mini-sized corncobs in some supermarkets – just right for babies. Corn is fun to eat, and babies love to hold and chew it.

Vegetables are good dipped in sauces and purées. Try using some of the recipes for vegetable purées as dipping sauces.

VEGETABLE VARIETY

beans (green), bell pepper, broccoli, butternut squash, carrots, cauliflower, celery, corncobs (and kernels and baby corn), eggplant, mushrooms, peas, potato, rutabaga, snowpeas, sweet potato, zucchini

Breads and Teething Biscuits

Pieces of toast, teething biscuits, and firm bread, like pita bread, can be dipped into purées and sauces. Often a baby who refuses to be spoon-fed will eat her meal by sucking it off a biscuit or piece of toast.

Many teething biscuits on the market contain as much sugar as a cookie and even so-called low-sugar ones can contain more than 15 percent sugar. It is very easy to make your own sugar-free alternative from wholewheat bread.

HOMEMADE TEETHING BISCUITS

For homemade teething biscuits, simply cut a thick (1/2 inch) slice of wholewheat (cracked wheat or rye) bread into three strips. Place on a cookie sheet and bake in the oven preheated to 350°F for 15 minutes. If your baby does not like plain teething biscuits, you could try adding a little grated cheese. If you wish, you could prepare a store of teething biscuits in advance. They will keep well in an airtight container for 3–4 days.

Rice cakes come in all different flavors and are excellent for teething, as they seem to hold together well.

Miniature Sandwiches

Little sandwiches cut into fingers, squares, small triangles, or even animal shapes using a cookie cutter are very popular with babies. Some suggestions for sandwich fillings are given below; see also the toddler section for a more exhaustive list (pages 186–187).

FILLING SUGGESTIONS

mashed banana, avocado and chopped tomato, tuna with corn and mayonnaise, cottage cheese and pineapple, cream cheese and strawberry jelly, Vegemite, grated cheese and tomato, mashed sardines with lettuce, egg mayonnaise and salad cress

---

Breakfast Cereals

Babies love to pick up and eat little pieces of breakfast cereal. Try to choose cereals that are fortified with iron and vitamins and which do not have any added sugar. Some suggestions for suitable cereals are given below.

GOOD MORNING MUNCHIES

Cheerios, Cornflakes, Granola, Chex, Grahams

Cheese

Start by giving your baby grated cheese or cut wafer-thin slices. Once she has mastered chewing, you can move on to chunks and strips of cheese. I have found that the following cheeses are especially popular: Cheddar, mozzarella, Edam, Swiss, and Monterey Jack. Cream cheese, ricotta, and cottage cheeses are also favorites. Avoid strong cheeses like blue cheese, Brie, and Camembert. Always make sure that the cheese you give your baby is pasteurized.

Pasta

Pasta comes in all shapes and sizes, it is soft to chew, and is very appealing to babies. I have given some recipes for pasta sauces but most of the vegetable purées can also be served with pasta. You can try tossing pasta in melted butter and sprinkling with grated cheese. This is usally a great favorite, even with the fussy eaters.

Meat

Slices or chunks of cooked chicken (or turkey) make great finger food for babies. As well as plain pieces of chicken, try giving your baby chicken cooked in a sauce. Very often the sauce makes the chicken more tender and so it is easier for your baby to chew.

Miniature chicken balls are another favorite (try my recipe for Chicken and Apple Balls, page 98). Your baby may also enjoy chewing on miniature drumsticks. Remove the skin and make sure that your baby avoids eating any pieces of bone. There is a fine needle-like bone in all drumsticks which is potentially very dangerous – extra care needs to be taken.

Strips of sautéed liver make good finger food as they are easy to hold and soft to eat. Try, too, some miniature meatballs (see page 154). Pieces of steak and chunks of meat are generally too tough for young babies to chew.

Fish

Pieces of flaked white fish are good as they are low in fat, high in protein, and easy for your child to chew. You can give them to your baby either plain or mixed with a sauce. Do take extra care, when serving fish to your baby in any recipe, to check the fish thoroughly for bones before you cook it and when flaking it.

Make your own fish fingers, fish balls, and fish cakes (see pages 94 and 133–34).

BREAKFAST

The first meal of the day is important to all of us after a night's fasting, particularly so for energetic babies and toddlers!

Recipes can now contain more interesting and more nutritious grains. Wheat-germ is particularly good and can be sprinkled on to cereals or yogurt. Mixing cereals and fruit makes a delicious and nutritious start to the day. Many of the homemade cereals can be mixed with apple juice instead of milk.

Cheese is important for strong bones and teeth. You can offer cheese on toast or little strips for your baby to hold. Eggs are an excellent source of protein, vitamins, and iron. Give your baby scrambled eggs or an omelet but make sure that the white and yolk are cooked until solid. Fresh fruit provides vitamins, minerals, and substances called phytochemicals, which help prevent cancer. Give fruit as finger foods, make fruit salads, or offer stewed fruit, such as apple or rhubarb.

Highly refined, sugar-coated cereals should be avoided. Do not be fooled by the list of added vitamins on the side of the box – unprocessed cereals are much healthier for your child.

There are also some recipes in the toddler baking and fruit dessert sections that make excellent breakfast food: Pineapple and Raisin Muffins (page 175), Funny Shape Cookies (page 172), or Snow-Covered Fruit Salad (page 165).

BREAKFAST

Fruity Swiss Muesli

This tasty and nutritious breakfast will make a good start to the day. You can vary the fruit in this muesli, adding, for example, peaches, strawberries, bananas, or chopped ready-to-eat dried apricots.

MAKES 4 ADULT PORTIONS

³/₄ cup regular oatmeal
³/₄ cup wheatgerm
³/₄ cup apple juice
1 teaspoon lemon juice

1 apple, peeled, cored, and grated
1 pear, peeled, cored, and chopped
1 tablespoon maple syrup
¹/₂ cup plain yogurt

Combine the oatmeal, wheatgerm, and apple juice. Set aside for a couple of hours or refrigerate overnight. Next morning, mix the lemon juice with the grated apple and stir this into the oat mixture together with the chopped pear, maple syrup, and yogurt.

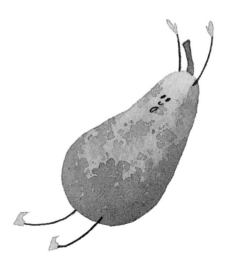

Fruity Yogurt

Many commercial fruit yogurts have a lot of added sugar. It is easy to make your own, adding a combination of your baby's favorite foods.

MAKES 2 ADULT PORTIONS

½ ripe peach, pitted, skinned, and chopped
½ small banana, peeled and chopped

⅝ cup plain yogurt
2 teaspoons maple syrup

Simply mix all the ingredients together and serve. Mash the fruit for younger babies.

☺ ☹

My Favorite Pancakes

Pancakes for breakfast are a treat, and this simple recipe is foolproof. Pancakes can be made in advance, refrigerated, and reheated. To freeze, interleave with non-stick baking paper. Serve with maple syrup and fresh fruit.

MAKES 12 PANCAKES

1 cup all-purpose flour
a good pinch of salt
2 eggs

1¼ cups milk
3 tablespoons melted butter

Sift the flour and salt into a mixing bowl, make a well in the center and add the eggs. Use a balloon whisk to incorporate the eggs into the flour and gradually whisk in the milk until just smooth.

Brush a heavy-based 6–7 inch skillet with the melted butter and, when hot, pour in about 2 tablespoons of the batter. Quickly tilt the pan from side to side to form a thin layer of batter and cook for 1 minute. Flip the pancake over with a spatula and cook until the underside is slightly golden. Continue with the rest of the batter, brushing the pan with melted butter when necessary.

☺ ☹ ❄

Apricot, Apple, and Pear Custard

Dried apricots are one of nature's great health foods. They are a good concentrated source of beta-carotene, potassium, and iron. This tasty fruit purée works well for breakfast or dessert.

MAKES 3 PORTIONS

½ cup ready-to-eat dried apricots
1 large dessert apple, peeled, cored, and chopped

1 tablespoon custard powder
¾ cup milk
1 ripe pear, peeled, cored, and chopped

Gently heat the apricots and apple in a small saucepan with 4 table-spoons water for 8–10 minutes or until soft. In another pan, blend the custard powder with a little of the milk to make a smooth paste. Then add the remaining milk and slowly bring to a boil, stirring until thickened and smooth. Blend the cooked fruit and pear to the desired consistency and stir in the custard.

A Grown-Up Breakfast

Unfortunately, many breakfast cereals designed specifically for children are laden with sugar. I give my children old-fashioned cereals like graham crackers, oatmeal, or muesli and sweeten them with fresh fruit.

MAKES 1 PORTION

1 tablespoon graham crackers
1 small banana

3 tablespoons plain yogurt or milk

Finely crumble the graham crackers and mash the banana. Combine all the ingredients and serve.

Summer Fruit Muesli

Simply soak the oatmeal overnight and stir in extra fresh fruits like peaches or strawberries the next day for a nutritious muesli. If your baby is too young for lumpy food, this can be blended to a fine purée.

MAKES 4 ADULT PORTIONS

1¹/₃ cups regular oatmeal
2 tablespoons golden raisins
1¹/₄ cups apple and mango juice
2 dessert apples, peeled, cored, and grated

4–6 tablespoons milk
a little maple syrup or honey (for babies over 1 year

Mix the oatmeal, golden raisins, and apple and mango juice in a bowl, cover, and leave to soak overnight in the refrigerator. In the morning, stir in the remaining ingredients and any extra fruit, and drizzle over a little maple syrup or honey (if using).

Banana and Prune Fool

This only takes a couple of minutes to prepare and is quite delicious. It is also a good recipe to try if your baby is a little bit constipated.

MAKES 1 PORTION

5 canned prunes in fruit juice, pitted
1 small ripe banana, peeled

1 tablespoon plain yogurt
1 tablespoon cream cheese

Place all the ingredients together in a blender with 1–2 tablespoons of the juice from the canned fruit. Blend until smooth.

The Three Bears' Breakfast

This makes a very nutritious breakfast, but make sure your child eats it up before Goldilocks comes to the front door!

MAKES 2 ADULT PORTIONS

1¼ cups milk
½ cup oatmeal

1 oz dried peaches or apricots, chopped
1 teaspoon raisins, chopped

Pour the milk into a saucepan and bring to a boil. Mix in the oatmeal and bring back to a boil, stirring. Add the chopped dried fruit, lower the heat, and simmer for about 4 minutes or until thickened.

Matzo Brei

For those of you who have never heard of *matzo*, it is a large square of unleavened bread similar to crispbread. When uncooked, it is very brittle and my son loved to snap it into pieces and strew it all over the floor. This is why I preferred to give it to him cooked!

MAKES 2 ADULT PORTIONS

2 matzos
1 egg, beaten

2 tablespoons butter
a little superfine sugar (optional)

Break the matzos into bite-sized pieces and soak for a couple of minutes in cold water. Squeeze out the excess water, then add the matzos to the beaten egg. Melt the butter in a skillet until sizzling and fry the matzos on both sides. Sprinkle with sugar if wished.

French Toast Cutouts

It's fun sometimes to cut the bread into a variety of animal shapes using cookie cutters. For a treat, serve with maple syrup or jelly.

MAKES 2 PORTIONS

1 egg
2 tablespoons milk
a pinch of powdered cinnamon (optional)

2 slices white or raisin bread
1½ tablespoons butter

Beat the egg lightly with the milk and cinnamon, if using, and pour into a shallow dish. Dip the bread in this mixture, coating each side. Melt the butter and fry the slices or animal shapes until golden on both sides.

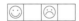

Cheese Scramble

Until your child is one year, scrambled egg should be cooked until it is quite firm and not runny. You could use cottage cheese instead of Cheddar.

MAKES 1 ADULT PORTION

1 egg
1 tablespoon milk
1 tablespoon butter

*1 tablespoon finely grated Cheddar
cheese*
1 tomato, skinned and seeded (optional)

Beat the egg with the milk. Melt the butter over a low heat and add the egg mixture. Cook slowly, stirring all the time. When the mixture has thickened and looks soft and creamily set, add the cheese and tomato. Serve immediately.

FRUIT

Baked Apples with Raisins

Tart apples have a better flavor but dessert apples are sweeter. You can use either for this recipe. The apples are delicious served with ice cream or custard sauce.

MAKES 6 BABY OR 2 ADULT PORTIONS

2 apples
½ cup apple juice or water
2 tablespoons raisins
a little powdered cinnamon

1 tablespoon maple syrup or honey (if using tart apples)
a little butter or margarine

Core the apples and prick the skins with a fork to stop them bursting. Put the apples in an ovenproof dish and pour the apple juice or water around the base. Put 1 tablespoon of the raisins into the center of each apple, sprinkle with cinnamon, and pour over the maple syrup or honey (if using tart apples). Top each with a little butter. Bake in an oven preheated to 350°F for about 45 minutes.

For young babies, scoop out the pulp of the apple and then purée coarsely with the raisins and some of the juices from the dish.

Apple and Blackberry

Blackberries and apples make a delicious combination, and the blackberries (which are rich in vitamin C) turn the apples a wonderful purple color. Instead of blackberries you could use other berry fruits like strawberries or blueberries, or a mixture.

MAKES 6 PORTIONS

2 tart apples, peeled, cored, and chopped

³/₄ cup blackberries
¹/₄ cup brown sugar

Cook the apples with the blackberries in a saucepan with the sugar and 1 tablespoon water. Cook until the apples are soft (15–20 minutes). Put the fruit through a mill to make into a smooth purée.

Rice Pudding with Peaches

MAKES 6 PORTIONS

1 tablespoon butter
¹/₃ cup short-grain rice
1 tablespoon each vanilla and brown sugar, or 2 tablespoons superfine sugar
2¹/₂ cups milk

1 teaspoon vanilla extract
1 heaped tablespoon raisins
a scant ¹/₂ cup peach juice
2 ripe peaches, skinned, pitted, and cut into pieces

Grease a shallow ovenproof dish with a little butter (a 1³/₄-pint oval Pyrex dish is ideal). Put the rice, sugar, milk, and vanilla extract into the dish and stir well. Dot with the remaining butter. Bake in an oven preheated to 300°F for about 2 hours, stirring after 30 minutes and again 30 minutes later. Meanwhile, simmer the raisins in the peach juice and purée the peaches. When the rice pudding is cooked, stir in the peach juice, raisins, and peach purée.

Fresh Pear with Semolina

This recipe is also good with apricots or apple purée with cinnamon. If you do not have any semolina, you can add a finely crushed rusk to the milk (which does not need to be boiled).

MAKES 2 PORTIONS

1 tablespoon semolina
½ cup milk
1 ripe pear, peeled, cored, and sliced

2 teaspoons maple syrup
a pinch of powdered cinnamon

Put the semolina and milk in a saucepan, bring to a boil, and simmer for 2 minutes. Add the pear, maple syrup, and cinnamon, then put all the ingredients through a mill to make a purée or chop the pear finely.

Strawberry Rice Pudding

The secret of a good rice pudding is long, slow, gentle cooking. It is good mixed with fruit purée like stewed apples and pears, stewed plums, or chopped canned peaches or apricots.

MAKES 6 BABY OR 3 ADULT PORTIONS

1 tablespoon butter
⅓ cup short-grain white rice
1–2 tablespoons superfine sugar

2½ cups milk
½ teaspoon vanilla extract
strawberry jelly, maple syrup, or honey

Grease a shallow ovenproof dish with a little butter. Put the rice and sugar into the dish, pour over the milk and vanilla extract and dot with a little butter. Bake in an oven preheated to 300°F for about 2 hours, stirring occasionally. Serve hot with strawberry jelly, maple syrup, honey, or fruit purée swirled into the rice.

Cheese and Raisin Delight

This makes a delicious combination and is very nutritious.

MAKES 2 PORTIONS

¼ cup Swiss cheese
½ apple, peeled and cored

1½ tablespoons raisins, chopped
1 tablespoon plain yogurt

Grate the Swiss cheese and apple and mix in the raisins and yogurt. For young babies who do not chew, put all the ingredients in a blender for about 1 minute. ☺ ☹

Dried Apricots with Papaya and Pear

Dried apricots are rich in beta-carotene and iron and they combine well with a variety of fresh fruits. This is also good mixed with yogurt. I found that my children also liked chewing on semi-dried apple rings, which are easy to hold because of the hole in the middle.

MAKES 4 PORTIONS

½ cup ready-to-eat dried apricots
½ ripe papaya, skinned, seeded, and chopped

1 ripe, juicy pear, peeled, cored, and chopped

Put the apricots in a small saucepan and just cover with water. Bring to a boil and simmer until softened (about 8 minutes). Drain and chop the apricots and mix with the chopped papaya and pear, or purée for babies who prefer a smoother texture. ☺ ☹ ❄

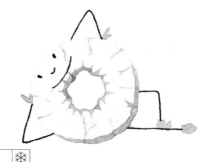

VEGETABLES

Risotto with Butternut Squash

Cooked rice with vegetables is nice and soft so it's a good way to introduce texture to your baby's food. Butternut squash is now more readily available in grocery stores and it is rich in vitamin A. You could use pumpkin to make this, instead of squash.

MAKES 3 PORTIONS

½ cup onion, chopped
1½ tablespoons butter
⅔ cup basmati rice
2 cups boiling water

5 oz butternut squash, peeled
and chopped
3 ripe tomatoes (about 8 oz), skinned,
seeded, and chopped
½ cup Cheddar cheese, grated

Sauté the onion in half the butter until softened. Stir in the rice until well coated. Pour over the boiling water, cover, and cook for 8 minutes over a high heat. Stir in the butternut squash, reduce the heat, and cook, covered, for about 12 minutes or until the water has been absorbed.

Meanwhile, melt the remaining butter in a small saucepan, add the chopped tomatoes, and sauté for 2–3 minutes. Stir in the cheese until melted. Add the tomato and cheese mixture to the cooked rice and combine. Season to taste for babies over one year.

Lentil and Vegetable Purée

This makes a delicious purée which my nine-month-old daughter loved.
Lentils are an excellent source of protein and very easy to cook.

MAKES 6 PORTIONS

2 tablespoons butter
1½ cups leek, washed and sliced
1½ cups carrot, chopped
¼ cup split red lentils

1½ cups vegetable broth (see page 33)
or water
1 cup cauliflower florets
½ dessert apple, peeled, cored,
and chopped

Melt the butter and sauté the leek for about 5 minutes. Add the carrot and continue to cook for 2–3 minutes. Add the lentils and broth, bring to a boil, then cover and simmer for about 15 minutes. Add the cauliflower and apple and cook for another 15 minutes or until the lentils and vegetables are tender. Purée to the desired consistency.

Multicolored Casserole

Babies love the bright colors and miniature size of these vegetables.
It makes eating fun, and is a good lesson in finger control.

MAKES 4 PORTIONS

1 tablespoon olive oil
1 shallot, peeled and finely chopped
a good ½ cup red bell pepper, diced

1 cup frozen peas
⅔ cup frozen corn kernels
½ cup vegetable broth or water

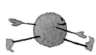

Heat the oil in a saucepan, add the shallot and red bell pepper, and cook for 3 minutes. Add the peas and corn, pour over the vegetable broth, and bring to a boil. Cover and simmer for 3–4 minutes.

Cabbage Surprise

This is a delicious recipe and very simple to prepare. It makes a great lunchtime meal for the whole family; just increase the quantities, sprinkle with extra grated cheese, either Cheddar or Parmesan, and brown under the broiler before serving. Alternately, mix all the cooked ingredients together and bake in the oven at 350°F for 15 minutes.

MAKES 6 PORTIONS

2½ tablespoons brown rice
1 cup cabbage, shredded
1 tomato, skinned, seeded, and chopped

a little butter
½ cup Cheddar cheese, grated

Cook the rice in water until quite soft (about 25 minutes). Boil the cabbage in water for about 5 minutes or until tender. Sauté the tomato in the butter, add the well-drained cabbage, and continue to cook for a further 2 minutes. Stir in the grated cheese and cook over a low heat until all the cheese has melted. Mix the cabbage, tomato, and cheese together with the cooked rice and chop it into small pieces.

Vegetables in Cheese Sauce

MAKES 6 PORTIONS

1 cup cauliflower florets
1 carrot, peeled and thinly sliced
½ cup frozen peas
1 zucchini (approx. 4 oz), washed
and sliced

Cheese Sauce
2 tablespoons butter
2 tablespoons all-purpose flour
1 cup milk
½ cup Cheddar cheese, grated

Steam the cauliflower and carrot for 6 minutes, then add the peas and zucchini and cook for a further 4 minutes. For a young baby, cook the vegetables until they are very soft.

Meanwhile, make the cheese sauce in the usual way (see page 59). Mash, chop, or purée the vegetables with the sauce.

Green Fingers

Green beans make great finger food and work well with this tasty sauce. Alternately, chop the beans into short lengths and mix with the sauce.

MAKES 2 PORTIONS

5 oz green beans, trimmed
1 small onion, peeled and finely chopped
1 tablespoon butter

2 medium tomatoes (8 oz), skinned,
seeded, and chopped
½ tablespoon tomato paste
¼ cup Swiss cheese, grated

Steam the beans for 6 minutes until tender. Sauté the onion in the butter for 4 minutes, add the tomatoes and tomato paste, and cook for 3 minutes. Place the beans in an ovenproof dish, cover with the tomato sauce, and sprinkle over the cheese. Place under a preheated broiler until the cheese is bubbling and golden.

FISH

Flounder with Herbs

Easy to make and all the flavor is sealed in a parcel.

MAKES 3 PORTIONS

1 fillet of flounder, skinned
1 teaspoon olive oil
1 small tomato, skinned, seeded,
and chopped

1 small zucchini, washed and sliced
2 teaspoons chives, chopped
1 sprig each of parsley, tarragon, and
chervil (optional)

Place the fish fillet on a piece of oiled aluminum foil. Mix all the remaining ingredients together and place on top of the fish. Wrap up securely. Cook in an oven preheated to 350°F for about 12 minutes or until the fish just flakes with a fork. Remove the herb sprigs and mash with a fork.

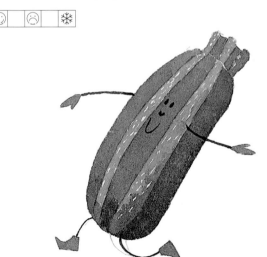

Fingers of Sole

These fingers of sole are fun for babies and toddlers to eat, and make great finger food. They can be served plain or, for older children, with a homemade tomato sauce. Simply purée 3 skinned and seeded tomatoes with a sautéed shallot, 1 tablespoon tomato paste, 2 teaspoons of milk, and a teaspoon of finely chopped basil. These "fish fingers" are much better for your child than commercial ones which are full of coloring and additives. If you are not using all the fingers at once, it is best to freeze them before they are cooked. You can then take out as many fingers as you need for a freshly cooked meal. You could substitute flounder for sole. Crushed cornflakes also make a delicious coating for other types of fish, such as haddock or cod.

MAKES 8 PORTIONS

1 shallot, peeled and finely chopped
1 tablespoon milk
1 tablespoon vegetable oil
1 sole, filleted and skinned

1 egg
all-purpose flour
crushed cornflakes
a little butter or margarine for frying

Mix together the chopped shallot, half the milk, and the oil. Marinate the fish fillets in this mixture for 1 hour. Remove the fillets from the marinade. Cut them into 4 or 5 diagonal strips, depending on the size of the sole. Beat the egg together with the remaining milk. Dip the strips first into the flour, then the egg and milk, and finally the crushed cornflakes. Fry the fingers in butter until golden brown on both sides. They should take no more than 5 minutes to cook.

Fillets of Sole with Grapes

Fillets of sole with grapes makes a delicious combination. This recipe is quick and easy to prepare and one that the whole family can enjoy.

MAKES 4 ADULT PORTIONS

8 single sole fillets
1 tablespoon seasoned flour
1¼ tablespoons butter
1 cup mushrooms, thinly sliced
a scant ½ cup fish broth

a scant ½ cup heavy cream
1 teaspoon lemon juice
2 teaspoons fresh parsley, chopped
20 seedless white grapes, halved
salt and pepper (for babies over one year)

Coat the fish with seasoned flour, melt half the butter in a large skillet, and fry the fish over a medium heat for about 2 minutes on each side until lightly golden. Transfer to a plate and keep warm.

Add the remaining butter to the pan and cook the mushrooms for 3 minutes. Add the broth and simmer for 2 minutes. Stir in the cream and lemon juice and then simmer for 2 minutes. Add the parsley and grapes, then season with salt and pepper (if using) and pour over the fish.

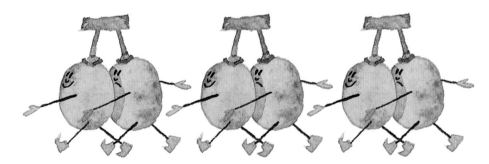

Gratin of Haddock with Tomato Sauce and Spinach

It is really important to encourage your baby to enjoy eating fish, and this is one of my favorite recipes – in fact, it's so good that the whole family enjoys it! Once cooked, the fish will just flake with a fork and will be nice and soft for your baby to eat.

MAKES 6 PORTIONS

1 tablespoon sunflower oil
½ cup onion, finely chopped
1 small garlic clove, crushed
1 cup passata (ready-strained tomatoes)
4 cups fresh spinach, washed and coarse stems removed

11 oz haddock or flounder fillets, skinned
2 tablespoons all-purpose flour
2 tablespoons butter
½ cup Cheddar cheese, grated

Heat the oil in a pan and sauté the onion and garlic until softened. Stir in the passata and cook over a medium heat for 2 minutes. Cook the wet spinach leaves in a pan, over a medium heat, for 3 minutes until just limp, then squeeze out the remaining moisture and chop coarsely. Coat the fish in flour, then melt the butter in a small skillet and sauté the fish for about one and a half minutes each side, until lightly golden and sealed.

Spread the spinach over the base of an ovenproof dish. Lay the fish on top, pour over the tomato sauce, and sprinkle over the grated cheese. Bake in an oven preheated to 350°F for 10 minutes or until the fish is cooked through. Flake the fish with a fork, and mix together with the spinach, tomato sauce, and cheese.

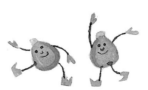

Salmon with a Creamy Chive Sauce

Salmon is easy to cook. It can be cooked very quickly in the microwave but here I have wrapped it in aluminum foil with some vegetables and herbs and cooked it more slowly to bring out the flavor.

MAKES 3 PORTIONS

4 oz fillet of salmon
2 teaspoons lemon juice
½ small onion, peeled and sliced
½ bay leaf
½ small tomato, cut into chunks
a sprig of parsley
a little butter

Chive Sauce
1 tablespoon butter
1 tablespoon all-purpose flour
½ cup milk
⅓ cup Cheddar cheese, grated
cooking liquid from the fish
2 teaspoons snipped chives

Wrap the salmon in aluminum foil with the rest of the ingredients and bake in an oven preheated to 350°F for 15 minutes. Meanwhile, make a thick white sauce, using the butter, flour, and milk in the usual way (see page 59). Stir in the Cheddar until melted.

Once the salmon is cooked, remove it from the foil, discard the onion, tomato, parsley, and bay leaf, strain off the cooking liquid, and add this to the white sauce. Finally, stir the snipped chives into the sauce. Flake the salmon and pour the chive sauce over it.

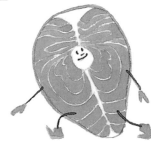

CHICKEN

Chicken with Couscous

MAKES 4 PORTIONS

1 tablespoon butter
¼ cup onion, chopped
¼ cup frozen peas, cooked

¾ cup chicken broth (see page 62)
⅜ cup quick-cooking couscous
2 oz chicken, diced and cooked

Melt the butter in a saucepan and sauté the onion until softened but not colored. Stir in the frozen peas, pour over the broth, bring to a boil, and cook for 3 minutes. Stir in the couscous, remove from the heat, cover, and set aside for 6 minutes. Fluff the couscous with a fork, and mix in the diced chicken.

☺ ☹ ❄

Chicken and Apple Balls

This is a great favorite with my family. Grated apple adds a delicious flavor to these chicken balls, which makes them appealing to young children and they are delicious hot or cold. These little balls make perfect finger food.

MAKES 20 CHICKEN BALLS

1 large dessert apple, peeled
and grated
2 large chicken breasts, cut into chunks
1 onion, peeled and finely chopped
½ tablespoon fresh parsley, chopped
1 tablespoon fresh thyme or sage,
chopped, or a pinch of mixed dried herbs

1 chicken bouillon cube, crumbled (for
babies over one year)
1 cup fresh white bread crumbs
salt and freshly ground pepper (for
babies over one year)
all-purpose flour for coating
vegetable oil for frying

Using your hands, squeeze out a little excess liquid from the grated apple. Mix the apple with the chicken, onion, herbs, bouillon cube (from one year), and bread crumbs and roughly chop in a food processor for a few seconds. Season with a little salt and pepper (from one year).

With your hands, form into about 20 little balls, roll in flour, and fry in shallow oil for about 5 minutes until lightly golden and cooked through.

Bang Bang Chicken

So called because my son likes to help when I flatten the chicken by banging it with a mallet! You can prepare these chicken fingers in advance. Before frying the chicken, cut it into strips, wrap each strip separately, and freeze. Just take one or two strips out of the freezer and fry them for freshly cooked chicken fingers.

MAKES 8 PORTIONS

1 double chicken breast, skinned and off the bone
3 slices white bread
1½ tablespoons grated Parmesan cheese (optional)

1 tablespoon fresh parsley, chopped (optional)
all-purpose flour for coating
1 egg, beaten
vegetable oil

Cover the chicken with waxed paper and flatten with a mallet or rolling pin, then cut each breast lengthwise into 4 strips. Make bread crumbs from the slices of bread in a food processor. If you are using the Parmesan and parsley, mix these together with the bread crumbs in a bowl.

Dip the chicken into the flour, then into the egg, and finally into the bread crumbs. Fry in oil for 3–4 minutes each side until golden on the outside and cooked through. Drain well on paper towels and then serve.

Chicken with Mashed Potato and Carrot

A good way to gradually introduce texture is to combine chopped food with creamy mashed potato – this can work well with chicken, meat, or fish.

MAKES 5 PORTIONS

1³/₄ cups potato, peeled and chopped
1³/₈ cups carrot, peeled and chopped
3 oz chicken, cut into chunks

1 cup chicken broth (see page 62)
2 tablespoons butter
3 tablespoons milk

Put the potato and carrot in a saucepan, pour over some boiling water, then cover and cook over a medium heat for 20 minutes or until the vegetables are tender. Meanwhile, poach the chicken in the broth for 6–8 minutes or until cooked through (allow to cool in the broth).

Drain the carrot and potato and mash together with the butter and milk. Chop the chicken into small pieces and serve with the mashed potato and carrot.

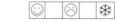

Chicken with Cornflakes

Cornflakes are very versatile, and I often use them instead of bread crumbs to coat both chicken and fish. These strips of chicken make good finger food. Before cooking, they can be individually wrapped and frozen.

MAKES 3–4 PORTIONS

1 egg, beaten
1 tablespoon milk
1 cup cornflakes, crushed

1 double chicken breast, skinned,
off the bone and cut into 8 strips
2 tablespoons butter, melted

Mix together the beaten egg and milk in a shallow dish. In a separate dish, spread out the cornflake crumbs. Dip the strips of chicken into the egg and then coat with the cornflakes. Put the chicken strips in a greased ovenproof dish, drizzle over the melted butter and toss to coat. Bake in an oven preheated to 350°F for about 10 minutes on each side or until cooked through. Alternately, the chicken strips can be sautéed in oil until golden and cooked through.

Chicken with Summer Vegetables

In the summer, you can often find different varieties of squash – some are round, some green, and some yellow. They are all delicious, but this recipe can also be made simply with zucchini.

MAKES 4 PORTIONS

1 small onion, chopped
1 garlic clove, crushed
¼ red bell pepper, seeded and finely chopped
1½ tablespoons olive oil
1 chicken breast, cut into chunks
2 tablespoons apple juice

¾ cup chicken broth (see page 62)
a small piece of yellow squash, chopped, or 1 large/2 small zucchini, finely chopped
1¾ cups sweet potato, peeled and chopped
1 tablespoon fresh basil, torn

Sauté the onion, garlic, and bell pepper in the olive oil until softened. Stir in the chicken and continue to cook for 3–4 minutes. Pour over the apple juice and broth and stir in the squash or zucchini, sweet potato, and basil. Bring to a boil, then cover and simmer for about 10 minutes. Chop or purée to the desired consistency.

Chicken with Winter Vegetables

This is quick and easy to prepare and has a delicious rich chicken flavor.
It is good with mashed potato.

MAKES 6 PORTIONS

*1 double chicken breast, on the bone
and skinned
a little flour
vegetable oil
1 small onion, peeled and finely chopped*

*1 white of leek, washed and sliced
1 carrot, peeled and sliced
1 celery stalk, trimmed and sliced
1¼ cups chicken broth
(see page 62)*

Cut the chicken breast into 4 pieces, roll each in flour, and brown them in a little oil for 3–4 minutes. In another skillet, sauté the onion and leek in a little oil for 5 minutes until soft and golden. Put the chicken into a Dutch oven together with all the vegetables and the broth. Cook in an oven preheated to 350°F for 1 hour, stirring halfway through.

Take the chicken off the bone and then chop the meat into little pieces with the vegetables, or purée it together with the cooking liquid in a mill or blender.

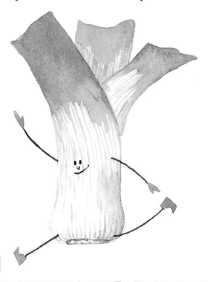

MEAT

Beef Casserole with Carrots

The secret for a delicious rich taste is to cook the meat for a long time so that it is very tender and has a good flavor from the onions and carrots. Increase the Vegemite for toddlers.

MAKES 6 PORTIONS

2 medium onions, peeled and sliced
vegetable oil
12 oz lean stewing beef, trimmed and cut into small chunks
2 medium carrots, peeled and sliced

1 beef bouillon cube, crumbled, or
1 teaspoon Vegemite (for babies over one year)
1 tablespoon fresh parsley, chopped
2½ cups water
2 large potatoes, cut into quarters

Fry the onions in a little oil until golden, then add the meat chunks and brown. Transfer the meat and onions to a small Dutch oven and add the rest of the ingredients except for the potatoes. Cook, covered, in an oven preheated to 350°F for 30 minutes, then turn down the heat and cook for a further 2½ hours at 325°F. One hour before you finish cooking the meat, add the potatoes.

Chop the meat quite finely in a food processor or blender so that it is easy for your baby to chew. If the meat gets too dry during cooking, add a little extra water. You can also add mushrooms and tomatoes to this recipe for variation. They should be added 30 minutes before the end of cooking time.

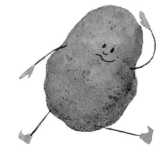

☺ ☹ ❄

Tasty Liver Casserole

Liver is very good for children: it is easy to digest, a good source of iron, and is very easy to cook. I must admit that I dislike the taste, having been forced to eat liver at school, but, to my great surprise, my one-year-old son adored it. This recipe is good served with mashed potato.

MAKES 4 PORTIONS

4 oz calf's liver, trimmed and sliced
2 tablespoons vegetable oil
1 small onion, peeled and chopped
1 large or 2 medium carrots (approx.
4½ oz), peeled and chopped

⅞ cup chicken or vegetable broth
2 medium tomatoes (approx. 7 oz),
skinned, seeded, and chopped
2 teaspoons fresh parsley, chopped

Sauté the liver in 1 tablespoon of the oil until browned, then set aside. Heat the remaining oil in a saucepan and sauté the onion for 2–3 minutes. Add the chopped carrot and sauté for 2 minutes, then pour over the broth, bring to a boil, cover, and simmer over a low heat for about 15 minutes. Chop the liver into pieces and add to the pan together with the tomatoes and parsley, and cook for about 3 minutes. You can either serve with mashed potato as it is or blend the mixture for a few seconds to make a coarse purée.

☺ ☹ ❄

Savory Veal Casserole

A delicious casserole of veal, vegetables, and fresh herbs – just increase the quantities for a meal the whole family can enjoy.

MAKES 3 PORTIONS

1 small onion, peeled and finely chopped
1 carrot, scraped and sliced
½ celery stalk, sliced
vegetable oil

4 oz lean veal for stewing
1 sprig rosemary
1 sprig parsley
½ cup water or chicken broth

Fry the onion, carrot, and celery in a little oil for 3 minutes. Cut the veal into chunks and put it into a saucepan with the vegetables, herbs, and water or broth. Simmer slowly, covered, for 1 hour, (stirring once). Remove the herbs and coarsely chop the veal and vegetables in a food processor.

Special Steak

This recipe makes a very good introduction to red meat for your baby.

MAKES 4 PORTIONS

1 potato (about 8 oz), peeled and chopped
1 shallot or ¼ cup onion, peeled and finely chopped
1 tablespoon vegetable oil

4 oz fillet steak
⅔ cup mushrooms, washed and chopped
1 tablespoon butter
1 tomato, skinned, seeded, and chopped
2 tablespoons milk

Boil the potato until tender, then drain. Meanwhile, sauté the shallot in the vegetable oil until softened. Spoon half the shallot onto a piece of aluminum foil. Cut the steak into slices ½ inch thick and place on top of the shallot. Spread the remaining shallot over the steak. Cook under a preheated broiler for 3 minutes each side or until cooked. Sauté the mushrooms in half of the butter for 2 minutes, add the tomato, and continue to cook for 1 minute. Mash the potato with the milk and remaining butter until smooth. Chop or purée the steak together with the shallot, mushrooms, and tomato, and mix with the mashed potato.

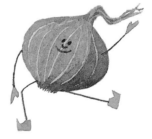

Mini Shepherd's Pie

Shepherd's pie was always a great "comfort food" on a winter's evening when I was a child. Try making small portions in ramekin dishes for your child. See page 155 for a more grown-up version.

MAKES 2–4 PORTIONS

1¾ cups potato, peeled and chopped
1 cup carrot, peeled and chopped
1 tablespoon olive oil
1 small onion, peeled and chopped
1 small garlic clove, peeled and crushed
½ cup red bell pepper, cored, seeded, and diced

⅝ cup (5 oz) lean ground beef
1 tablespoon fresh parsley, chopped
1 teaspoon tomato paste
a scant ½ cup chicken broth (see page 62)
a little butter
1 tablespoon milk

Put the potato and carrot into a saucepan, cover with boiling water, and cook until the vegetables are tender (about 20 minutes).

Meanwhile, heat the oil in a skillet and sauté the onion, garlic, and bell pepper for 2–3 minutes. Add the ground beef and sauté until browned. At this stage, chop the meat in a food processor for a few seconds to give it a smoother texture. Return to the pan, add the parsley, tomato paste, and chicken broth, bring to a boil, then cover and simmer for about 15 minutes.

When the potato and carrot are cooked, drain and mash together with some of the butter and the milk until smooth. Mix with the meat and spoon into small (4-inch) ramekin dishes. Heat through in an oven preheated to 350°F, then dot with the remaining butter and place under a preheated broiler until lightly golden.

Tasty Rice with Meat and Vegetables

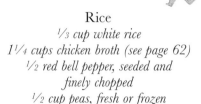

MAKES 6 PORTIONS

½ onion, peeled and finely chopped
1 carrot, peeled and finely chopped
vegetable oil
1 cup lean ground beef
½ tablespoon tomato catsup
a few drops of Worcestershire sauce

Rice
⅓ cup white rice
1¼ cups chicken broth (see page 62)
½ red bell pepper, seeded and
finely chopped
½ cup peas, fresh or frozen

Put the rice into a saucepan and cover with the chicken broth. Bring to a boil, then cover and simmer for 15 minutes. Add the red bell pepper and peas and cook, uncovered, for 6–7 minutes, or until the rice is tender and there is no liquid left.

Meanwhile, sauté the onion and carrot in a little vegetable oil for 5 minutes. Add the ground meat and cook, stirring, until browned. Stir in the tomato catsup and Worcestershire sauce and cook over a gentle heat for 10 minutes. Chop the meat in a food processor for about 30 seconds to make it easier for your baby to chew.

Put the meat into a saucepan, stir in the rice (with the chicken broth), and cook over a gentle heat for 3–4 minutes.

PASTA

Salmon and Broccoli Tagliatelle

Pasta is popular with babies and toddlers, so combining it with nutritious foods like salmon and broccoli is a good idea.

MAKES 6 PORTIONS

3 cups tagliatelle
1 small carrot
³/₄ cup broccoli, cut into small florets
1¹/₄ cups milk
1 bay leaf
3 peppercorns

a sprig of fresh parsley
5 oz fillet of salmon, skinned
1 tablespoon butter
¹/₈ cup flour
¹/₂ teaspoon lemon juice
¹/₂ cup Cheddar cheese, grated

Cook the tagliatelle according to the packet instructions. Steam the broccoli or cook in boiling water for about 4 minutes or until tender. Pour the milk into a saucepan together with the bay leaf, peppercorns, and parsley, and bring to a boil. Reduce the heat, place the salmon in the pan, and simmer covered for 6–8 minutes or until the fish is just cooked. Remove the salmon with a slotted spoon and strain the milk.

Melt the butter, stir in the flour, and cook for 1 minute. Gradually whisk in the reserved milk. Bring to a boil and then simmer for 2 minutes. Stir in the lemon juice and cheese until melted.

Flake the fish and stir into the cheese sauce together with the broccoli cut into small pieces. Chop the tagliatelle into short lengths and mix with the cheese sauce.

☺ ☹ ❄

My Favorite Bolognese

MAKES 6 PORTIONS OF SAUCE

2 tablespoons vegetable oil
1 large onion, peeled and chopped
1 large carrot, grated
1½ cups mushrooms, sliced
1½ cups beef broth
1 garlic clove, crushed
2 cups lean ground beef
1 cup passata (ready-strained tomatoes)

1 tablespoon tomato paste
1 tablespoon tomato catsup
½ tablespoon Worcestershire sauce
1 bay leaf
½ teaspoon mixed dried herbs
salt and freshly ground black pepper (for babies over one year)

Heat 1 tablespoon of the vegetable oil in a saucepan, and sauté half the onion for 3 minutes, stirring occasionally. Add the carrot and mushrooms and sauté for 5 minutes more. Transfer to a blender, stir in ½ cup of the beef broth, and blitz until smooth.

Meanwhile, heat the remaining oil in a saucepan and sauté the garlic and remaining onion for 3 minutes. Add the ground beef and sauté, stirring occasionally, until browned. Add the remaining broth, the rest of the ingredients, and the carrot and mushroom mixture. Bring to a boil and simmer, uncovered, for 15–20 minutes. Remove the bay leaf and serve.

Pasta Stars with Tomato and Cheese

The fresh tomato sauce is very tasty and, because it has vegetables and cheese blended into it, it is more nutritious than an ordinary tomato sauce.

MAKES 2 PORTIONS

1 medium carrot, peeled and sliced
1 cup cauliflower florets
3 tablespoons pasta stars or other tiny pasta shapes

1½ tablespoons butter
11 oz ripe tomatoes, skinned, seeded, and chopped
½ cup Cheddar cheese, grated

Put the sliced carrot into the bottom of a steamer. Cover with boiling water and cook over a medium heat for 10 minutes. Put the cauliflower florets in the steamer basket, place over the carrot, cover, and cook for 5 minutes or until the vegetables are tender. Cook the pasta stars in boiling water according to the packet instructions. Meanwhile, melt the butter and sauté the tomatoes for about 3 minutes or until mushy. Stir in the Cheddar cheese until melted. Blend the cooked carrot and cauliflower together with the tomatoes and cheese. Mix with the pasta stars.

Pasta Shells with Tuna and Corn

Tuna is a good store-cupboard standby. It is rich in protein, vitamin D, and vitamin B12.

MAKES 3 PORTIONS

½ cup small pasta shells or other small pasta shapes
1½ tablespoons butter
2 tablespoons flour

1¼ cups milk
⅜ cup Swiss cheese, grated
4 oz canned tuna, drained and flaked
½ cup canned or cooked frozen corn kernels

Cook the pasta according to the packet instructions. Melt the butter in a saucepan. Add the flour and stir in for about 1 minute. Slowly add the milk, stirring continuously until the sauce has thickened. Stir in the cheese, tuna, corn, and pasta and heat through.

Tuna Salad

Oily fish like tuna and salmon contains omega-3 fatty acids, which help prevent heart disease and are important for brain and visual development. Unfortunately, fatty acids are destroyed in the canning process of tuna but you could make this salad using fresh tuna or salmon instead.

MAKES 4 PORTIONS

1½ cups cooked pasta butterflies or shells
1 scallion, finely chopped, or
1 small shallot, peeled and diced
⅔ cup canned tuna in oil, drained and flaked
3 cherry tomatoes, quartered
¼ cup canned corn kernels (or cooked frozen corn)
1 small avocado, peeled, pitted, and cut into small pieces (optional)

Dressing
1 tablespoon mayonnaise
1 tablespoon olive oil
1 teaspoon fresh lemon juice

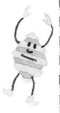

Mix together the ingredients for the dressing. Combine the cooked pasta with the salad ingredients and toss with the dressing. If you wish, toast some sesame seeds in a dry skillet until golden and sprinkle these on top (see page 138).

NINE-TO-TWELVE-MONTH MEAL PLANNER

	Breakfast	Mid-morning	Lunch
Day 1	**Fruity Swiss Muesli** **Dried Apricots with Papaya and Pear** served with yogurt Milk	Milk	**Chicken and Apple Balls** Finger vegetables **Strawberry Rice Pudding** Water
Day 2	Chex (or other cereal) Cheese on toast Fruit Milk	Milk	**Special Steak** **Homemade Fruit Gelatin** Fruit Water
Day 3	Scrambled egg and toast Fruit with cottage cheese Milk	Milk	**Pasta Shells with Tuna and Corn** Water
Day 4	**My Favorite Pancakes** Fruit Milk	Milk	**Tasty Liver Casserole** **Multicolored Casserole** Papaya purée Water
Day 5	**French Toast Cutouts** **Apricot, Apple, and Pear Custard** Milk	Milk	**Bang Bang Chicken** **Cabbage Surprise** **Homemade Fruit Gelatin** Fruit Water
Day 6	**Summer Fruit Muesli** Yogurt with dried fruit Milk	Milk	**Beef Casserole with Carrots** **Going Bananas** Water
Day 7	**Cheese Scramble** Toast fingers **Fruity Yogurt** Milk	Milk	**Chicken with Couscous** **Fresh Pear with Semolina** Water

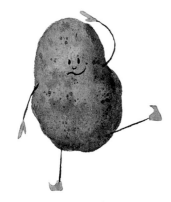

Mid-afternoon	Dinner	Bedtime
Milk	Finger sandwiches Finger vegetables Juice or water	Milk
Milk	**Pasta Stars with Tomato and Cheese** Yogurt Juice or water	Milk
Milk	**Zucchini and Pea Soup** Fruit Juice or water	Milk
Milk	**Vegetables in Cheese Sauce** **Apple and Blackberry** Juice or water	Milk
Milk	**Tomato and Zucchini Pasta Stars** Fruit Juice or water	Milk
Milk	**Fingers of Sole** Finger vegetables **Rice Pudding with Peaches** Juice or water	Milk
Milk	**Lentil and Vegetable Purée** Sticks of cheese **Baked Apples with Raisins** Juice or water	Milk

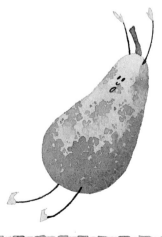

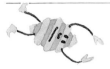

CHAPTER FIVE

TODDLERS

I find that beyond the age of one, toddlers prefer to exercise their independence and feed themselves. The more your toddler experiments using a spoon and fork, the quicker he will master the art of feeding himself – you never know, some food might find its way into his mouth! A "pelican" bib – a strong plastic bib that has a tray at the bottom to catch stray food – is also good. If your toddler has difficulty eating with a spoon, try giving him finger foods, such as sautéed strips of fish or raw vegetables, with a dip. You must still be careful, though, to keep food like olives, nuts, or fresh litchis out of the reach of young children. Toddlers love to put everything in their mouths and it would be so easy for them to choke on such foods.

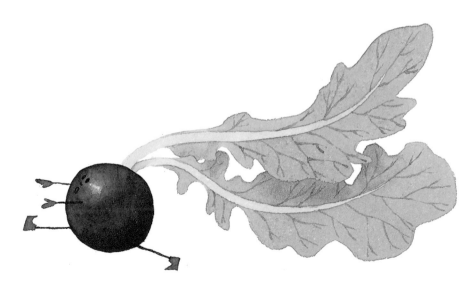

ENJOYING MEALTIMES TOGETHER

Toddlers only have small tummies and often can't eat enough at mealtimes to fuel their high energy requirements, so they should be offered three meals and three snacks at regular times. There is a whole section in this book on healthy snacks, so don't make the mistake of giving your toddler candy or processed snacks when he could enjoy eating a dip with a bowl of raw vegetables. Toddlers who get accustomed to eating healthy snacks are more likely to continue the same habits later on in life. However, it would also be wrong to make candy and doughnuts the forbidden fruit, or your toddler would crave them all the more and possibly gorge himself on them whenever he is out of the house.

Many toddlers enjoy eating much more sophisticated food than we would imagine possible. Let your child try food from your plate and you may find yourself very surprised by the tastes he enjoys. Of course food from Mommy's or Daddy's plate is much more interesting than his own meal and you can sometimes entice your child to eat better if you put his meal on your plate. But the point at this stage is that the toddler can now eat, to a large extent, what you adults are eating. I am a great believer in giving toddlers "grown-up" foods as soon as possible, and almost all the recipes that follow are suitable for the whole family. *Do* eat with your child rather than just sitting there shoveling food into his mouth. He'll eat much more happily *with* you – after all, who enjoys eating alone?

Try and reform your own eating habits by adding less salt and sugar to your food, and your toddler will be able to enjoy almost everything you cook. I hope that you will enjoy many happy mealtimes together and that your children will introduce you to some great new recipes!

MY CHILD WON'T EAT!

After the age of one, your child will be expending much more energy, and nearly all toddlers at some stage will lose interest in food and would much rather play with their toys and run around. This can be a very difficult time and it is important not to make a big fuss if your child refuses to eat. He will eat when he is hungry and the more you fuss, the more he will refuse his food. Be patient with him – he will grow out of this phase.

If your toddler really enjoys his food and eats well at mealtimes, then you really are a lucky mother. I know so many mothers who worry constantly that their child is not eating enough. The majority of these worries are unnecessary, and toddlers can thrive very well on remarkably little food. Toddlers are very unpredictable: some days they will be ravenous, and other days they will eat practically nothing at all. If you judge your child's food intake over a whole week rather than just one day, you won't worry as much if one day he refuses to eat anything.

Many mothers complain that their toddler will not touch meat or fish but there are lots of other equally good sources of protein, such as peanut butter, eggs, or dairy produce. Then there are the mothers who are tearing their hair out because their children will only eat one thing. This is also quite normal: children, unlike adults, like repetition in their diet and they are often wary of trying new foods.

Avoid the empty calories found in cookies, cakes, and candy and, instead, offer healthy alternatives like fruit or raw vegetables such as carrot and cucumber with a tasty dip or cheese. Don't give drinks just before a meal as this can spoil your baby's appetite.

Unfortunately, over the past 50 years children's consumption of cookies has risen fourfold, confectionery by 25 times and soft drinks by 34 times. Meanwhile, the consumption of milk, bread, fruit, and vegetables has declined. The processed foods and ready meals that are now popular are high in saturated fat, salt, and sugar. It is very important to make sure that children eat as much fresh food as possible. One in four children in the US is overweight and the number of obese children has doubled in the last 20 years.

By this age your child is probably quite independent and may well prefer to feed himself. Toddlers enjoy playing with their food; it's all part of the learning process. Let your toddler eat spaghetti with his hands and poke his finger into the gelatin to see it wobble – there is plenty of time to teach him table manners once he has finished experimenting. Let your child help prepare meals – this may well stimulate an interest in food. My son is always willing to lend a helping hand, especially when it comes to making cookies. He loves to knead the dough, roll it out, and cut it into shapes. He thinks it's more fun than play dough!

A great deal of problem eating can be overcome by attractive presentation. Choose foods that are naturally brightly colored. It is a good idea to use plastic plates with separate compartments and present your toddler with two or three foods in separate sections. We have little Chinese meals at home and you can buy plastic chopsticks that are joined at the top, which even a three-year-old can use. You should see how they enjoy picking the food up with their chopsticks and how wide they open their mouths!

Sometimes it is fun to arrange food in a pattern on the plate. You can help teach your child by arranging food in the shape of numbers or letters or make the food into the shape of a face. You can use some small-sized novelty cookie cutters to cut out shapes from bread, sandwiches, or cheese to stimulate your child's interest. Another tip is to call food by funny names like Bugs Bunny carrots or Mickey Mouse soup. You may laugh but if your toddler thinks this is what his favorite character eats for lunch, he is more likely to eat it himself.

Never put too much food on a plate; it is much better that your child should ask for more. Toddlers love individual portions of food. Make a miniature casserole, for example, which is much nicer than a dollop of meat and potatoes on a plate, and miniature cakes rather than offering a slice from a large cake.

If you have given your toddler a good choice of foods and he still refuses to eat, it is not, then, a good idea to offer him the contents of the refrigerator and pantry. Explain that this is his meal and that there

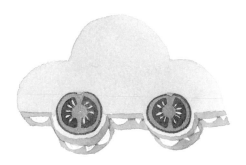

is nothing else on offer. If he is very restless and clearly not interested in eating, just put the food back in the refrigerator and bring it out again a little later. Toddlers will only eat when they are hungry – and no child has ever starved to death through stubbornness.

For breakfast, give your child oatmeal or Chex rather than sugar-coated cereals, and offer toast with peanut butter or Vegemite rather than toast and jelly. Cheese on toast and well-cooked scrambled eggs

are other healthy breakfast options. For supper, chicken on the griddle is a good alternative to chicken nuggets, give fish pie rather than fish sticks, pasta with broccoli or homemade tomato sauce rather than spaghetti hoops, homemade burgers instead of frozen burgers, and shepherd's pie instead of sausages and French fries. For snacks, give popcorn instead of potato chips, and dried fruit like apricots or yogurt-covered raisins instead of candy. Give juice or smoothies that are 100 percent fruit juice instead of fruit-juice drinks, which often contain less than 10 percent juice and lots of sugar and water.

If you make eating fun, then your child will be tucking in with you. An occasional trip to a restaurant does wonders to stimulate a child's appetite. Even just going to a friend's house for supper can help sometimes, especially if there is another child present who likes to eat!

THE FOODS TO CHOOSE

Children under the age of five need more dietary fat than adults in proportion to their body weight, so unless your child is overweight, do not give him foods that are low fat. Fat is a rich source of energy and fat-soluble vitamins, which your toddler needs in order to grow. There are, of course, exceptions to the rule, and an overweight toddler should have his fat intake restricted by cutting down on processed and fatty foods, and switching to low-fat dairy products.

High-fiber foods in large amounts are also unsuitable as they are bulky and filling and do not supply enough calories for a rapidly growing toddler. Also, a high- fiber diet can hinder the absorption of vital minerals like iron. Provided your child eats plenty of fruit and vegetables he will get all the fiber he needs.

Once your child is twelve months old, you can switch from formula to whole cow's milk, but don't give low-fat milk before the age of two as it is low in energy, which your child needs to grow. Skim milk should not be introduced before 5 years. Children over one year need 14 fl oz (1³/₄ cups) of whole milk a day. For children who are very picky, there may be advantages to continuing with a follow-on formula (which is fortified with vitamins and iron) until two years of age.

Although more and more people seem to be turning away from red meat in favor of fish and chicken, bear in mind that red meat provides more iron and zinc than

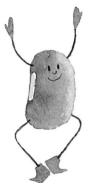

either fish or poultry. Try making tasty meals with lean ground meat – a good tip is to cook the meat and then chop it in a food processor so that it is not lumpy, and there are some lovely recipes for beefburgers, meatballs, and shepherd's pie (see pages 153–55) that make excellent family meals.

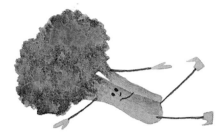

Try to avoid processed meats like sausages, salami, and corned beef.

If you are bringing your child up on a vegetarian diet, or if he simply dislikes eating meat, make sure that you include nutrient-dense foods like cheese and eggs in his diet. Provided your toddler is eating a good variety of food types, a vegetarian diet can provide all the nutrients he needs. It is very important to include vegetarian sources of iron such as green vegetables, pulses, fortified breakfast cereals, and dried fruit every day, and make sure you give foods or drinks containing vitamin C at the same meal as this helps to boost the iron in non-meat sources.

Pasta remains a great favorite with toddlers and you can combine it with other healthy foods such as vegetables and tuna. Individual pieces of pasta like penne or fusilli tend to be easiest for toddlers to eat. (Although, when my son Nicholas was 20 months old, he invented his own method of eating spaghetti – he held it out in front of him by the two ends and sucked in from the middle! Not the height of good manners perhaps, but certainly very efficient.)

Fruit and Desserts

There are many recipes in this chapter for delicious hot and cold desserts that are easy to prepare and can be enjoyed by the whole family. However, there is still nothing more delicious and better for you than fresh, ripe fruit, so make sure your child has plenty of it every day. None of the vitamins or nutrients are destroyed through cooking, and fruit makes great finger food for your toddler.

Fruits are packed with powerful antioxidants and natural compounds called phytochemicals, which help boost immunity and protect the body from heart disease and cancer. The incidence of cancer is increasing. Approximately one third of cancer cases are related to what we eat, and researchers estimate that a diet filled with fruit and vegetables instead of fats and processed foods, along with exercise, could reduce the incidence of cancer by at least 30 percent.

Whole fruit in a fruit bowl isn't that appealing to a hungry child, but if you have a selection of fresh fruit cut up and placed on a low shelf in the refrigerator, this will help stop your child from snacking on potato chips or cookies.

Dried fruits, especially apricots, are very nutritious as the drying process concentrates the nutrients. However, take care not to give dried fruit too often in between meals, as they stick to the teeth, and even natural sugars cause tooth decay.

Kiwi fruit and citrus and berry fruits are rich in vitamin C, which helps to boost iron absorption, so try to make sure you include these in your child's diet. You can add fresh or dried fruits to breakfast cereals. It's also a good idea to buy a juicer so that you can make your own fresh-fruit smoothies. Pure fruit juice and smoothies are also good, but be wary of fruit-juice drinks as they often contain as little as 10 percent juice so always read the label. Juices are a good source of vitamins, but remember that only by eating the whole fruit will your child be getting fiber.

As different fruits provide different nutrients, include as much variety as possible in your child's diet. Try introducing

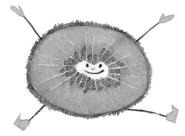

him to some more exotic fruits. One kiwi fruit contains more than the daily adult requirement of vitamin C and makes a good snack when cut in half, placed in an egg cup, and eaten with a teaspoon. You could also make a tropical fruit salad with mango, melon balls, pineapple, and a sauce made with fresh orange juice and passion fruit.

You can make delicious and healthy suckers from puréed fresh fruits, yogurt, fruit juices, or smoothies. Sucker molds are cheap to buy, and one food that almost no child can resist is a sucker, so this is a good way to encourage children to eat more fruit.

Ice creams in all colors, shapes, and sizes are sold all over the world. However, the quality of some products is put to shame by the genuine, homemade experience. If you do buy ice creams, choose those that are made from natural ingredients only. If you want to try your hand at making your own, it really is worth investing in an ice-cream-making machine, which churns the mixture as it freezes. Believe me, you will put it to good use over the years and your children will be very popular with their friends when they come round for supper.

Baking for Toddlers

A toddler's first birthday is a big occasion in his life and probably even more exciting for his parents and grandparents! It is great fun preparing the food for a child's party. Anyone can call a store and order a birthday cake in the shape of a train, but how much more impressive and satisfying it is to bake and decorate your own. Your child will love to help with the mixing and decorating, which are probably more fun than eating the cake.

Any basic sponge or fruitcake mixture could be adapted to a novelty shape, if you like. There are many smaller cakes that can be served at a child's party. Many of the baking recipes contain healthy ingredients, cutting out undesirables as much as possible, and some are sheer, uncompromised treats.

Healthy Snacks

If your toddler is happy to eat three main meals a day, then that is wonderful and very convenient for everyone, but let's face it, nearly all toddlers snack between meals. Whereas for some this just supplements their meals, many toddlers do not have the patience to sit down and eat a proper meal and they get most of their nutrition from snacks eaten during the day. Toddlers' stomachs are small and it is often difficult for them to eat enough at breakfast, say, to last them until lunchtime when they have been rushing around all morning. As I said earlier, lots of small meals – healthy snacks – during the day are in fact healthier than three main meals. Snacks are therefore a very important part of your toddler's diet. If you encourage your child when he is very young to enjoy eating healthy snacks in preference to candy and potato chips, it is likely that he will continue these habits later in life and enjoy a much healthier diet.

Stock your pantry and refrigerator with healthful snacks (see pages 180–81) and, when you take your toddler out, try to remember to take a small bag of healthy snacks with you. Toddlers expend a lot of energy and it doesn't take them long to get hungry again after a meal.

TEXTURES AND QUANTITIES

There is no longer any need to purée your child's food; on the contrary, he should be getting used to chewing. The longer you continue with purées because that is the way your child prefers his food, the more difficult it will become to encourage him to chew and swallow his food properly. In fact, chewing on something hard, such as a raw carrot, should help to relieve sore gums. A lot of toddlers, however, do not like to chew chunks of meat, and it is sometimes necessary to break meat down in a blender before serving it. I find that ground meat, liver, or chicken tends to go down better with most toddlers than chunks of meat.

With each recipe in this chapter, I have given quantities in adult portions. Every child is different, and you must judge the portion size according to your toddler's appetite. He can eat anything from one-quarter of an adult portion to a whole portion if he is very hungry and greedy!

OVERWEIGHT TODDLERS

In the US, one in ten children under the age of five is overweight, and 13 percent of all children are obese. If your child is overweight, then you should discuss with your doctor the best ways of decreasing his calorie intake. Adopt a healthier eating plan rather than cutting down on the amount of food offered. No child should ever go hungry. Cut out sugary, fatty, and processed foods and give more fresh fruit and vegetables. Give high-fiber cereals like Chex or Bran Flakes, give baked potatoes instead of French fries, and broiled or roast chicken instead of chicken nuggets. Low-fat milk can be introduced from two years.

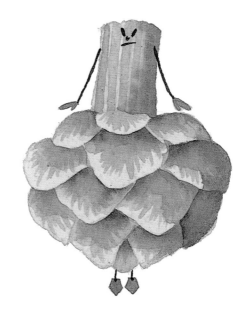

VEGETABLES

Ratatouille with Rice or Pasta

Vegetables tend to be quite soft in ratatouille and so are easy for your toddler to chew. Choose a firm eggplant and zucchini; if they are not fresh, the ratatouille may taste bitter. Serve as an accompaniment to a meal with rice, as below, or with pasta shapes. It is suitable for freezing without the rice.

MAKES 4 ADULT PORTIONS

2 tablespoons olive oil
1 red onion, peeled and chopped
1 garlic clove, peeled and crushed
1 small red bell pepper and 1 small green bell pepper, seeded and diced
1 zucchini, trimmed and diced
1 small eggplant, trimmed and diced
14 oz canned chopped tomatoes

pinch of sugar
1 teaspoon red wine vinegar
salt and pepper

Rice
1 vegetable bouillon cube
1 bay leaf
1 cup long-grain rice

Heat the oil in a large saucepan and cook the onion and garlic for 1–2 minutes. Add the bell peppers and zucchini and cook for 4–5 minutes. Add the eggplant and cook for 5 minutes. Stir in the chopped tomatoes, sugar, and red wine vinegar, bring to a simmer, and then cook for 10 minutes. Season with salt and pepper.

For the rice, place the vegetables, crumbled bouillon cube and bay leaf in a large saucepan of water. Stir in the rice and cook according to the packet instructions.

☺ ☹

Special Fried Rice

Babies love rice and this is very appealing as it is so colorful. For older children, you can make little sailing boats. Cut a cooked red bell pepper in half, stuff each half with rice, and stick two corn chips upright in the rice to look like sails.

MAKES 6 ADULT PORTIONS

1¼ cups basmati rice
¾ cup carrot, diced
¾ cup frozen peas
¾ cup red bell pepper, seeded and diced
2 eggs, lightly beaten

3 tablespoons vegetable oil
1 small onion, peeled and finely chopped
1 scallion, finely sliced
1 tablespoon soy sauce
salt

Wash the rice thoroughly and cook according to the packet instructions in a saucepan of lightly salted water until tender. Steam the carrot, peas, and bell pepper for 5 minutes or until tender. Heat 1 tablespoon of the oil in a skillet. Season the eggs with a little salt, add to the pan, tilting it so the eggs form a thin layer over the bottom, and fry until set like a very thin omelet. Remove from the skillet and cut into thin strips. Meanwhile, put 2 tablespoons of oil into a wok or skillet and sauté the chopped onion until softened. Add the rice and vegetables and cook, stirring, for 2–3 minutes. Add the egg and scallion and cook, stirring, for 2 more minutes. Sprinkle with the soy sauce before serving.

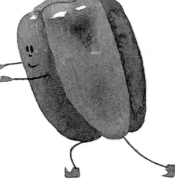

Stuffed Potatoes

Stuffed potatoes make an excellent meal for toddlers and there are endless variations on the fillings you can make. Prick medium potatoes all over and brush with oil. Bake in an oven preheated to 375°F for 1¼–1½ hours, or until tender. Alternately, to speed up the cooking, prick the potatoes, wrap them in absorbent kitchen paper, and put them in the microwave on high for 7–8 minutes. Brush the potatoes with oil and then transfer to the oven and cook for about 45–50 minutes or until tender.

Carefully spoon the soft flesh out of the skins, leaving enough round the sides for the skins to keep their shape. You are now ready to make the various fillings.

Vegetable and Cheese Potato Filling

MAKES 4 ADULT PORTIONS

¼ cup each of small broccoli and cauliflower florets
4 medium or 2 large baked potatoes
1 tablespoon butter
½ cup milk

½ cup Cheddar cheese, grated
2 medium tomatoes, skinned and cut into small pieces
¼ teaspoon salt
grated cheese to finish

Steam the cauliflower and broccoli until tender (about 6 minutes) and then chop finely. Meanwhile, mash the potato flesh with the butter and milk until smooth and creamy. Mix in the cheese, tomatoes, cooked chopped vegetables, and salt, and scoop the mixture back into the potato skins. Sprinkle a little extra grated cheese on top and then brown under a preheated broiler.

☺ ☹ ❄

Tuna and Corn Stuffed Potato

Other good fillings are scallion and bacon with sour cream, and
vegetarian chilli with cheese.

MAKES 2 ADULT PORTIONS

2 medium baked potatoes
2 tablespoons mayonnaise
2 tablespoons milk
1 cup Cheddar cheese, grated

salt and pepper
5 oz canned tuna in oil, drained
3 oz canned or cooked frozen corn kernels
1 scallion, finely sliced (optional)

Cut the baked potatoes in half and scoop out the flesh, leaving enough
around the sides for the skins to keep their shape. Mash the potato
flesh together with the mayonnaise, milk, and $1/2$ cup of the grated cheese,
and season to taste with a little salt and pepper. Stir in the flaked tuna,
corn, and scallion (if using). Spoon the filling back into the potato skins,
place on a cookie sheet, and scatter over the remaining grated cheese.
Place under a preheated grill for about 2 minutes or until golden.

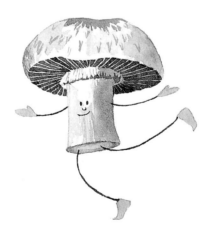

Stuffed Tomatoes

Another easy dish, which can be prepared in advance and which looks very appealing.

MAKES 2 ADULT PORTIONS

2 eggs
2 medium tomatoes
1 tablespoon mayonnaise

1 tablespoon snipped chives
salt and pepper

Hard-boil both the eggs. Meanwhile, skin the tomatoes, then cut the tops off and scoop out the insides. Discard the seeds but keep the tiny bits of flesh. When the eggs are ready, peel and mash them together with the pieces of tomato, mayonnaise, chives, and a little salt and pepper. Stuff into the tomatoes and replace the tomato tops on the egg mixture.

Delicious Vegetable Rissoles

Nuts and tofu are great for vegetarians as they contain many of the nutrients usually found in animal sources. Tofu and cashew nuts are both excellent sources of protein and iron.

MAKES 10 RISSOLES

1¼ cups carrot, grated
1 medium zucchini (approx. 4½ oz),
topped, tailed, and grated
1 scant cup leek, finely chopped
1 garlic clove, crushed
2½ cups mushrooms, chopped
1½ tablespoons butter
7 oz firm tofu, chopped into pieces

½ cup unsalted cashew nuts,
finely chopped
2 cups fresh, white bread crumbs (made
from sliced bread)
1 tablespoon soy sauce
1 tablespoon runny honey
salt and pepper
flour for coating
vegetable oil for frying

Prepare the vegetables and, using your hands, squeeze out any excess liquid from the grated carrot and zucchini. Melt the butter in a skillet and sauté the leek, garlic, carrot, and zucchini for 2 minutes. Add the mushrooms and cook, stirring occasionally, for 2–3 minutes.

Add the tofu, cashew nuts, bread crumbs, soy sauce, honey, and seasoning, mix well and form into 10 rissoles. Coat in flour and sauté in the oil for about 2 minutes on each side, until golden.

Carrot and Zucchini Fritters

These are quick and easy to make. They are a good way to encourage your child to eat more vegetables and also make a delicious accompaniment to a family meal.

MAKES 4 ADULT PORTIONS

3 oz carrot, peeled
3 oz zucchini, trimmed
3 oz potato, peeled
1 medium onion, peeled
3 tablespoons ground almonds

2 tablespoons all-purpose flour
2 tablespoons lightly beaten egg
salt and pepper to taste
vegetable oil for frying

Grate the carrot, zucchini, potato, and onion. Cup small handfuls of the grated vegetables in the palm of your hand and squeeze out the excess moisture. Put the vegetables in a bowl and mix with the almonds, flour, and egg. Season to taste. Using your hands, form into 6 round, flat cakes and sauté in vegetable oil until golden on both sides and cooked through (about 6 minutes).

My Favorite Spanish Omelet

This is good served cold and cut into wedges the next day. I also give some suggestions for additions to the basic omelet.

MAKES 4 ADULT PORTIONS

3 tablespoons olive oil
6 oz potato, peeled and cut
into ½ inch cubes
1 onion, peeled and finely chopped
½ small red bell pepper, seeded
and chopped
½ cup frozen peas
4 eggs
2 tablespoons grated Parmesan cheese
salt and pepper

Suggested Variations
2 tablespoons Swiss cheese, grated,
instead of Parmesan
1 large tomato, skinned, seeded,
and chopped
OR
⅔ cup mushrooms, sliced
1 tablespoon chives, snipped
OR
⅔ cup cooked ham or bacon, cubed
⅓ cup corn kernels instead of peas

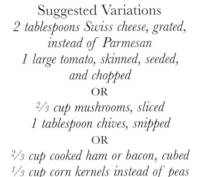

Heat the oil in a nonstick 7-inch skillet. Fry the potato and onion for 5 minutes, then add the bell pepper and cook for a further 5 minutes. Add the peas and continue to cook for 5 minutes. Beat the eggs together with 1 tablespoon water and the Parmesan, and season with salt and pepper. Pour this mixture over the vegetables and cook for 5 minutes or until the omelet is almost set. To finish, brown under a hot broiler for about 3 minutes or until golden. (You can wrap the handle of the skillet with foil to prevent it burning if necessary.) Cut into wedges and serve hot or cold with salad.

Annabel's Hidden-Vegetable Tomato Sauce

This is the perfect recipe for children who won't eat their vegetables, as all the vegetables are blended into the tomato sauce so they can't be identified or picked out. This tasty sauce can be used as a topping for pizzas or as a sauce for chicken and rice.

MAKES 4 ADULT PORTIONS

2 tablespoons light olive oil
1 garlic clove, crushed
1 medium onion, peeled and finely chopped
1 cup carrot, peeled and grated
$\frac{1}{2}$ cup zucchini, grated
$\frac{2}{3}$ cup mushrooms, sliced
1 teaspoon balsamic vinegar

$1\frac{3}{4}$ cups passata (ready-strained tomatoes)
1 teaspoon soft brown sugar
1 vegetable bouillon cube dissolved in a good $1\frac{1}{2}$ cups boiling water
a handful fresh basil leaves, torn
salt and freshly ground black pepper

Heat the oil in a saucepan, add the crushed garlic, and sauté for a few seconds, then add the onion and sauté for a further 2 minutes. Add the carrot, zucchini, and mushrooms and sauté for 4 minutes, stirring occasionally. Add the balsamic vinegar and cook for 1 minute. Stir in the passata and sugar, cover, and simmer for 8 minutes. Add the vegetable broth and cook for 2 minutes, stirring continuously. Add the basil and season to taste. Transfer to a blender and blitz until smooth.

Vegetable Salad with Walnut and Raspberry Vinegar

This is a refreshing salad for a summer's lunch. The dressing complements the nutty flavor of the corn and adds a little sweetness to the salad.

MAKES 4 ADULT PORTIONS

1 cup cauliflower florets
1 cup green beans, sliced
1 cup canned or frozen corn kernels
sugar and salt to taste
1/4 small crisp lettuce, shredded
8 cherry tomatoes, cut in half

1 hard-boiled egg, grated

Dressing
1 tablespoon raspberry vinegar
3 tablespoons walnut or hazelnut oil
salt and pepper to taste

Steam the cauliflower and beans until tender (about 10 minutes). Cook the frozen corn for about 4 minutes in boiling water with a little sugar and salt. When the cauliflower, beans, and corn have cooled, put all the salad ingredients in a bowl with the grated egg sprinkled on top. Mix the dressing ingredients together with a fork and pour over the salad.

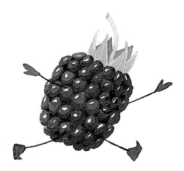

My Favorite Pasta with Broccoli

This is very simple and quick to prepare, and it is a great favorite with my three children.

MAKES 4 CHILD PORTIONS

1¾ cups fusilli pasta
1½ cups broccoli, cut into florets
1½ tablespoons butter
½ tablespoon sunflower oil

1 onion, peeled and finely chopped
1 garlic clove, peeled and crushed
1 chicken bouillon cube, dissolved in
½ cup boiling water

Cook the pasta according to the packet instructions. Steam the broccoli for 4 minutes, then set aside. Heat the butter and oil in a wok and sauté the onion and garlic for 3 minutes. Add the steamed broccoli and stir-fry for 1 minute. Stir in the chicken broth, add the cooked, drained pasta and heat through.

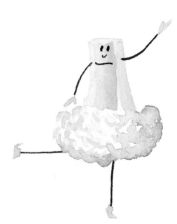

Mini Pizzas with Puff-Pastry Base

Ready-rolled puff pastry from the grocery store makes a good base for these delicious individual pizzas. You can vary the toppings, maybe adding extras such as mushrooms, ham, or pepperoni.

MAKES 4 INDIVIDUAL PIZZAS

1 tablespoon tomato paste
1 tablespoon olive oil
pinch of mixed dried herbs
salt and pepper to taste
12 oz ready-rolled puff pastry

4 scallions, trimmed and sliced
4 tablespoons frozen corn kernels
2 slices salami or pepperoni, cut into thin strips, (optional)
1⅛ cups mozzarella cheese, cubed

Place the tomato paste, olive oil, and mixed dried herbs in a small saucepan. Season with salt and pepper. Bring to a boil and simmer for 5 minutes until thickened. Cut four 6-inch circles out of the pastry (you could cut around a saucer) and place these on an oiled cookie sheet. Using a sharp knife, score a circle ¼ inch from the edge of the pastry to form a rim.

Divide the tomato mixture between the pastry bases and spread evenly. Sprinkle over the scallions, corn, and salami (if using), and top with the mozzarella cheese. Season with salt and pepper. Bake in an oven preheated to 350°F for 16–18 minutes.

FISH

Grandma's Gefilte Fish

This is my mother's traditional recipe. It is very appealing to children because of the slightly sweet taste of the balls. My son, Nicholas, loves them and they are very easy for him to hold and eat himself. Adults can eat them with horseradish sauce.

MAKES ABOUT 20 BALLS

1 onion, peeled and very finely chopped in the food processor
2 tablespoons butter
1 lb minced fish fillet (mix any of the following: haddock, halibut, whitefish, cod, or flounder)

1 egg, beaten
1 tablespoon sugar
salt and pepper to taste
light cooking oil for frying

Sauté the onion in the butter until lightly golden. Add to the remaining ingredients and mix well. Shape into golf-ball-sized balls. Fry carefully until golden brown all over. Drain on paper towels. Serve hot or cold.

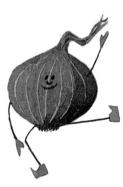

Salmon Fishcakes

Salmon is a good source of omega-3 fatty acids, which are important for brain and visual development. Doctors recommend including at least two oil-rich fish dishes a week to keep the heart in good shape. These fishcakes taste good hot or cold.

MAKES 8 FISHCAKES

*11 oz potato, peeled and cut
into chunks
1 tablespoon butter
14 oz canned red salmon, drained
½ small onion, peeled and finely chopped
2 scallions, finely chopped*

*2 tablespoons tomato catsup
salt and pepper
flour for coating
1 egg, lightly beaten
1½ cups matzo meal or bread crumbs
oil for frying*

Boil the potato in a saucepan of lightly salted water. Drain and mash with the butter. Flake the salmon and carefully remove any bones. Mix with the mashed potato, onion, scallions, tomato catsup, and seasoning. Form into about 8 fishcakes, coat in flour, dip in the egg, and then coat in matzo meal or bread crumbs. Heat the oil in a large skillet and fry the fishcakes until golden.

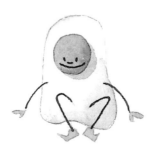

Nursery Fish Pie

A good, old-fashioned favorite.

MAKES 3 ADULT PORTIONS

12 oz haddock fillet, skinned, or 6 oz
each of haddock and salmon fillets
1½ cups milk
1 bay leaf
4 peppercorns
a sprig of fresh parsley
salt and pepper
1½ tablespoons butter
¼ cup all-purpose flour
⅜ cup Cheddar cheese, grated
2 tablespoons chives, snipped

½ tablespoon dill weed, chopped
(optional)
2 teaspoons lemon juice
1 hard-boiled egg, chopped
½ cup frozen peas, cooked following
packet instructions

Topping
1¼ lb potato, peeled and cut into pieces
2 tablespoons butter
2 tablespoons milk

Put the fish in a saucepan with the milk, bay leaf, peppercorns, parsley, and seasoning. Bring to a boil, then simmer, uncovered, for about 5 minutes or until the fish is cooked. While the fish is cooking, cook the potato for the topping in boiling, lightly salted water until soft. Drain well, then mash together with 1½ tablespoons of the butter and the milk.

Drain the fish, reserving the cooking liquid. Melt the butter in a heavy-based saucepan and stir in the flour. Cook gently for 1 minute, then whisk in the fish liquid gradually and bring to a boil. Simmer the sauce for 2–3 minutes until smooth, stirring continuously. Take off the heat and stir in the grated cheese until melted. Break the fish into chunks and fold in together with the chives, dill weed (if using), lemon juice, boiled egg, peas, and seasoning. Place the fish in an ovenproof dish (a 7 inch-diameter and 3 inch-deep, round dish is perfect) and top with the mashed potato. Bake in the oven preheated to 350°F for 15–20 minutes. Dot with the remaining butter and broil for about 2 minutes until brown and crispy.

Fish in Creamy Mushroom Sauce

For older children, cook 4 cups fresh spinach and lay each whole fillet on a bed of spinach and pour over the sauce.

MAKES 4 ADULT PORTIONS

*1 small onion, peeled and
finely chopped
3 tablespoons butter
3 cups mushrooms, finely chopped
2 tablespoons lemon juice*

*1 tablespoon parsley, chopped
2 tablespoons all-purpose flour
1¼ cup milk
1 x 7 oz sole (or flounder), filleted*

Fry the onion in half the butter until translucent. Add the mushrooms, lemon juice, and parsley and cook for 2 minutes. Add the flour and cook for 2 minutes, stirring constantly. Add the milk gradually and cook, stirring constantly, until the sauce is thick and smooth.

Fry the sole fillets in the rest of the butter for 2–3 minutes on each side. Cut or flake the fish into small pieces and mix with the mushroom sauce. Alternately, cover the fish with the mushroom sauce and bake in an oven preheated to 350°F for about 15 minutes or until the fish just flakes.

Gratin of Sole

A very tasty fish recipe which is so easy to make.

MAKES 4 ADULT PORTIONS

*4 fillets of sole or flounder
salt and pepper to taste
½ small lemon
2 cups wholewheat bread crumbs*

*½ cup Cheddar cheese, grated
1 heaped tablespoon parsley, chopped
¼ cup margarine, melted*

Lay the fillets in a greased ovenproof dish and season with salt, pepper, and lemon juice. Put the bread crumbs, cheese, and parsley in a bowl and stir in the melted margarine. Put the bread crumb mixture on top of the fish in the dish. Place the fish under a preheated broiler for about 8 minutes until the bread crumbs have turned a golden brown and the fish is cooked.

Cod in a Cheese Sauce with Matchstick Vegetables

Cod is particularly delicious roasted in the oven, and here it is served with colorful strips of vegetables and a tasty cheese sauce.

MAKES 2 ADULT PORTIONS

¼ red bell pepper, cut into thin strips
¼ yellow bell pepper, cut into thin strips
½ onion, peeled and thinly sliced
1 small zucchini, cut into matchsticks
1 tablespoon olive oil
2 x 7 oz cod or haddock fillets, skinned

salt and pepper
1 tablespoon butter
⅛ cup flour
1 cup milk
⅜ cup Swiss cheese, grated
⅜ cup mature Cheddar cheese, grated

Place the vegetable matchsticks in a small roasting tin, drizzle over the olive oil, and cook in the oven preheated to 350°F for 10 minutes, turning occasionally. Season the fish with salt and pepper and place on top of the vegetables. Return to the oven and cook for a further 10 minutes.

For the sauce, melt the butter in a saucepan and stir in the flour. Cook for 1–2 minutes, then gradually whisk in the milk. Simmer for 2–3 minutes. Stir in the grated cheeses until melted. Arrange the vegetables on a plate with a portion of fish on top and pour over some of the cheese sauce.

Chinese-Style Fish Fingers

Although rare, children can be allergic to sesame seeds. Take care, particularly if your child has other food allergies or conditions like eczema or asthma.

MAKES 1 ADULT PORTION

*2 x 5 oz fillets of flounder or sole,
skinned
all-purpose flour
2 tablespoons butter*

*1 teaspoon sesame seeds
1 tablespoon minced scallions
1 tablespoon soy sauce
2 tablespoons orange juice*

Coat the fish in flour and sauté for 2 minutes in the butter with the sesame seeds. Add the remaining ingredients and cook over a low heat for 2–3 minutes or until cooked.

☺ ☹

Salmon and Potato Mash

Salmon is a good source of essential fatty acids, which are important for brain and visual development.

MAKES 2 ADULT PORTIONS

*2³/₄ cups peeled, diced potato
5 oz salmon fillet, skinned
2 tablespoons butter*

*2 ripe tomatoes, skinned, seeded,
and chopped
2 tablespoons milk*

Put the potato in the bottom of a steamer, add boiling water, cover, and cook for 6 minutes. Place the salmon in the steamer over the potato, cover, and cook for another 6 minutes. Meanwhile, melt half the butter and sauté the tomato for 2–3 minutes. Drain the potato and mash together with the remaining butter and milk. Flake the salmon, mix with the tomato, and season to taste with salt and pepper. Serve with the mashed potato on the side.

☺ ☹

Grandma's Tasty Fish Pie

This is one of my mother's recipes which is a great favorite with all the family. There is never any left the next day.

MAKES 6 ADULT PORTIONS

1 lb skinned fillets of haddock or cod
salt and pepper
all-purpose flour
1 egg, beaten
2 slices wholewheat bread or 1 crisp roll, made into bread crumbs
cooking oil
1 onion, peeled and finely chopped
1 small red and 1 small green bell pepper, seeded and chopped

14 oz canned tomatoes, or 2 tablespoons tomato paste

Cheese Sauce
2 tablespoons margarine
1 tablespoon all-purpose flour
1 cup milk
$^3/_4$ cup Cheddar cheese, grated
$^3/_8$ cup Parmesan cheese, grated

Dip the fish fillets into seasoned flour, then into the egg, and finally coat in bread crumbs. Fry in oil until golden brown on both sides. Drain off the oil on paper towels, then flake the fish into small pieces and place in an ovenproof dish.

Sauté the onion in a very little oil in a skillet for 3–4 minutes. Add the bell peppers and continue to cook until soft. Drain the can of tomatoes, chop the tomatoes, and add to the bell peppers and onion (or simply add the tomato paste). Cook for 3–4 minutes, then season. Pour over the fish.

Make a cheese sauce with the margarine, flour, and milk, stirring over a low heat until smooth and thick (see page 59). Take the saucepan off the heat and stir in two-thirds of the Cheddar and Parmesan, reserving the rest to sprinkle over the top of the fish pie.

Cover the flaked fish and tomato with the cheese sauce and top with the reserved grated cheese. Cook in an oven preheated to 350°F for 20 minutes. Brown under the broiler.

Kids' Kedgeree

This is a really scrummy kedgeree, which makes a great family meal that is popular with kids. It's the kind of food you could eat for breakfast or supper. If you want to make a smaller amount, simply halve the quantities.

MAKES 6 ADULT PORTIONS

12 oz undyed smoked haddock
a scant $\frac{1}{2}$ cup heavy cream
$1\frac{1}{2}$ tablespoons butter
1 onion, peeled and chopped
1 teaspoon mild curry paste

1 cup basmati rice, cooked
1 teaspoon lemon juice
2 tablespoons fresh parsley, chopped
2 hard-boiled eggs, chopped
salt and pepper

Place the haddock in a microwave-proof dish and pour over the cream. Cover with saran wrap, pierce a few times with the tip of a sharp knife, and place in the microwave on High for 5–6 minutes. Meanwhile, in a skillet or wok, melt the butter and sauté the onion for 8 minutes until soft. Stir in the curry paste and rice and cook for 1 minute, stirring continuously. Flake in the haddock and add the cooking liquid, lemon juice, parsley, and chopped eggs. Season with salt and pepper if necessary.

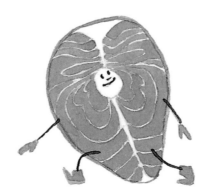

Toasted Tuna Muffins

A can of tuna in the pantry is a good standby and tuna is rich in protein, vitamin D and vitamin B12. These toasted muffins are quick and easy to make for a tasty and healthy meal.

MAKES 1–2 PORTIONS

4 oz canned tuna in oil, drained
1 tablespoon mayonnaise
1 tablespoon tomato catsup
1 scallion, finely chopped

2 tablespoons canned corn
kernels (optional)
1 English muffin
¼ cup Cheddar cheese, grated

Flake the tuna into a bowl and stir in the mayonnaise, tomato catsup, scallion, and corn (if using). Preheat the broiler, divide the muffin into 2 halves and toast. Divide the tuna mixture between the 2 halves. Cover with the grated cheese and place under the broiler for about 2 minutes until golden and bubbling.

Tuna Pita Pocket

MAKES 2 PITA POCKETS

4 oz canned tuna in oil, drained
⅓ cup corn kernels
1 hard-boiled egg, chopped
1 tablespoon mayonnaise
½ teaspoon white wine vinegar

2 scallions, chopped
1 tomato, skinned, seeded, and chopped
salt and freshly ground black pepper
1 pita bread

Flake the tuna with a fork and mix with the corn, hard-boiled egg, mayonnaise, white wine vinegar, scallions, tomato, and seasoning. Toast the pita bread, cut in half to make two pockets, and divide the mixture between them.

Tuna Tagliatelle

This is my favorite tuna recipe.

MAKES 6 ADULT PORTIONS

½ onion, peeled and finely chopped
2 tablespoons butter
1 tablespoon cornstarch
½ cup water
14 fl oz canned cream of tomato soup
a pinch of mixed dried herbs
1 tablespoon fresh parsley, chopped
7 oz canned tuna, drained and flaked
black pepper
3 cups green tagliatelle
1 tablespoon Parmesan cheese, grated

Mushroom Cheese Sauce
½ onion, peeled and finely chopped
2 tablespoons butter
1½ cups mushrooms, washed and sliced
2 tablespoons all-purpose flour
1¼ cups milk
1 cup Cheddar cheese, grated

For the sauce, fry the onion in the butter until transparent, then add the sliced mushrooms and sauté for about 3 minutes. Add the flour and continue stirring the mixture all the time. When it is well mixed, add the milk gradually and cook, stirring until thickened and smooth. Remove from the heat and stir in the grated cheese.

Fry the onion in the butter until soft. Stir the cornstarch into the water until dissolved, and mix with the tomato soup. Add the mixed dried herbs and fresh parsley and cook, stirring, over a low heat for 5 minutes. Mix in the flaked tuna and heat through. Season with a little black pepper.

Boil the tagliatelle in water until *al dente*, then drain. Grease a serving dish and add the tuna and tomato mixed with the pasta and then the mushroom cheese sauce. Top with grated Parmesan. Bake in an oven preheated to 350°F for 20 minutes. Brown under a hot broiler before serving.

Tuna with Pasta and Tomatoes

Most children like penne with tomato sauce, and it's a good idea to add some canned tuna and grated cheese to boost the nutritional content. Semi-dried sunblush tomatoes add a lovely flavor to this dish.

MAKES 6 ADULT PORTIONS

2 cups penne (tubes)
2 tablespoons olive oil
1 medium red onion, peeled and chopped
1 garlic clove, crushed
½ small red bell pepper, cored, seeded, and chopped
1½ cups mushrooms
28 oz canned chopped tomatoes

4 oz sunblush tomatoes, chopped
14 oz canned tuna in sunflower oil, drained
2 teaspoons balsamic vinegar
½ teaspoon mixed dried herbs
a handful fresh basil leaves, torn
1¼ cups Cheddar cheese, grated

Cook the penne according to the packet instructions. In a large saucepan, heat the oil and sauté the onion, garlic, and red bell pepper for 5 minutes, stirring occasionally. Add the mushrooms and cook for a further 3 minutes. Add the canned tomatoes, sunblush tomatoes, flaked tuna, balsamic vinegar, and dried herbs and cook for 10 minutes uncovered. Stir in the drained, cooked pasta and the fresh basil.

Transfer to a fairly shallow ovenproof dish and sprinkle with the grated cheese. Preheat the broiler on a high setting and cook for about 3 minutes or until golden and bubbling.

CHICKEN

Thai-Style Chicken and Noodles

Don't be afraid to try out new tastes on your child – this recipe flavored
with mild curry and coconut sauce is very popular. Young children often
surprise us and like quite sophisticated foods and it's usually easier to get
children to accept new tastes while they are young. This would make a
good meal for the whole family.

MAKES 4 PORTIONS

Marinade
1 tablespoon soy sauce
1 tablespoon sake
½ teaspoon sugar
1 teaspoon cornstarch

1½ chicken breasts cut into strips
¾ cup Chinese noodles
1 tablespoon vegetable oil
3 scallions, sliced

1 garlic clove, crushed
*½ teaspoon red chilli, seeded
and chopped*
1½–2 teaspoons korma curry paste
⅝ cup chicken broth (see page 62)
⅝ cup coconut milk
6 baby corncobs, cut into quarters
1½ cups bean sprouts
¾ cup frozen peas

Mix together the ingredients for the marinade and marinate the chicken
for at least 30 minutes. Cook the noodles according to the packet
instructions, drain, and rinse under cold water. Heat the vegetable oil in a wok
or skillet and stir-fry the scallions, garlic, and chilli for about 2 minutes. Drain
the marinade from the chicken, add to the wok, and continue to stir-fry for
2 minutes. Add the curry paste, chicken broth, and coconut milk and cook
for 5 minutes over a low heat. Add the baby corncobs and bean sprouts and
cook for 3–4 minutes. Finally, add the peas and cook for 2 minutes more.

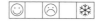

Bar-B-Q Chicken

A good marinade will transform your barbecue, tenderizing the meat as well as adding a delicious flavor. I use a Weber Bar-B-Q, which has a cover, thus enabling me to barbecue food all year round. Use 2 lb breast of chicken, skinned and on the bone, with these marinades – they also work well with beef or lamb.

MAKES 4–5 ADULT PORTIONS

Hoisin Marinade
2 tablespoons soy sauce
2 tablespoons hoisin sauce
2 tablespoons rice wine vinegar
1 tablespoon honey
1 tablespoon vegetable oil
½ teaspoon minced garlic (optional)

Teriyaki Marinade
3 tablespoons red wine vinegar or white wine vinegar
2 tablespoons soy sauce
1 tablespoon honey
½ tablespoon sesame oil
1 teaspoon grated ginger root (optional)
1 tablespoon sliced scallion

Mix all the marinade ingredients together. Marinate the chicken for at least 2 hours, then barbecue, basting and turning occasionally, for 15–25 minutes – dark meat takes longer to cook than white meat. The chicken should be cooked through but not overcooked or it will become dry. If you are unsure about cooking chicken thoroughly before the surface is charred, cook it in an oven preheated to 400°F for 25–30 minutes and finish it on the barbecue for a few minutes to give an authentic flavor.

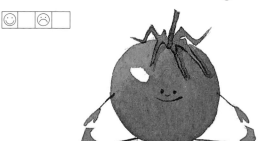

Chicken Satay

These barbecued chicken skewers are fun to eat and very popular with toddlers. Help your child take the meat off the skewers and then remove the skewers – they could become dangerous in the hands of exuberant toddlers.

MAKES 2 ADULT PORTIONS

*2 double chicken breasts, off the bone
and skinned
1 small onion, peeled
1 small red bell pepper, seeded
8 mushrooms, washed*

Marinade
*2 tablespoons peanut butter
1 tablespoon chicken broth (see page 62)
1 tablespoon rice wine vinegar
1 tablespoon honey
1 tablespoon soy sauce
1 teaspoon minced garlic (optional)
1 teaspoon sesame seeds, toasted
(optional, see page 131)*

In a bowl, mix together all the ingredients for the marinade. Soak 4 bamboo skewers in water to prevent them getting scorched. Cut the chicken, onion, and bell pepper into chunks. Leave the chicken in the marinade for at least 2 hours. Thread the chicken, onion, bell pepper, and mushrooms onto the skewers, then barbecue, basting the chicken frequently with the marinade.

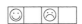

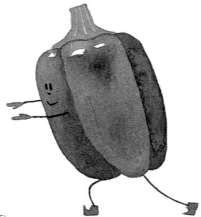

Peanuts can cause allergic reactions (see page 15).

Chicken Soup with Pasta and Vegetables

This is a very quick and easy chicken noodle soup that is very popular with my three children. Vermicelli is very fine pasta that comes rolled up in nests.

MAKES 6 PORTIONS

4 cups chicken broth
1 tablespoon vegetable oil
1 onion, peeled and thinly sliced
1 garlic clove, crushed
4½ oz chicken breast, cut into bite-sized pieces

¼ teaspoon chicken seasoning
½ cup green beans, topped, tailed, and cut into short lengths
¾ cup vermicelli or ⅓ cup tiny pasta stars
1 tomato, skinned, seeded, and chopped

Make up the chicken broth in a pan using either 2 chicken bouillon cubes and boiling water, liquid broth from a supermarket, or my recipe on page 62. Meanwhile, heat the vegetable oil in another saucepan and sauté the onion and garlic for 2 minutes. Add the chicken, sprinkle with chicken seasoning, and sauté for 1 minute, stirring occasionally, then add the green beans and sauté for 3 minutes. Mix the chicken, onion, green beans, and vermicelli with the chicken broth. Bring to a boil, then reduce the heat, and cook for 3–4 minutes or until the pasta is cooked and the beans are just tender. Stir in the chopped tomato and cook for 1 minute.

Chicken Fillets with Mango Chutney and Apricot

This is very simple to prepare but tastes absolutely delicious. It is a great favorite with children because of the sweet and sour taste.

MAKES 2 ADULT PORTIONS

1 double chicken breast, off the bone and skinned

Sauce
1 tablespoon apricot jam
1 tablespoon mango chutney
3 tablespoons mayonnaise
1 teaspoon Worcestershire sauce
1 tablespoon lemon juice

Mix all the ingredients together for the sauce. Put the chicken into a small ovenproof dish, pour over the sauce, and cover the dish with aluminum foil. Bake in an oven preheated to 350°F for 30 minutes.

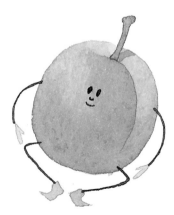

Stir-Fried Chicken with Vegetables and Noodles

Stir-fries are popular with children and make great family food. To save time you could try using a pack of ready-prepared stir-fry vegetables from the grocery store and then just add a few extra favorite vegetables of your own.

MAKES 4 ADULT PORTIONS

Marinade
1½ tablespoons soy sauce
1 tablespoon sake
1 teaspoon sesame oil
1 tablespoon white wine vinegar
1 teaspoon soft brown sugar
1 teaspoon cornstarch

2 skinless chicken breasts, cut into strips
⅔ cup fine Chinese egg noodles
3 tablespoons vegetable oil

1 onion, peeled and finely sliced
1 garlic clove, peeled and crushed
¾ cup carrot, cut into matchsticks
6 baby corncobs, cut into quarters
¾ cup broccoli, cut into florets
1 cup zucchini, trimmed and cut into matchsticks
1½ cups bean sprouts
1 chicken bouillon cube, dissolved in ¾ cup boiling water
salt and freshly ground black pepper

Mix the marinade ingredients and marinate the chicken for at least 30 minutes. Cook the noodles according to the packet instructions, then drain and stir in a little oil to prevent them sticking. Strain the marinade from the chicken and reserve. Heat 1 tablespoon of the oil in a wok and stir-fry the chicken for 4–6 minutes until cooked through, then set aside. Heat the remaining oil in the wok and sauté the onion and garlic for 3 minutes. Add the carrot, baby corncobs, and broccoli and stir-fry for 3 minutes. Add the zucchini and bean sprouts and stir-fry for 2 minutes. Pour the chicken broth into a small saucepan and add the reserved marinade. Bring to a boil, stirring until thickened. Season with a little salt and pepper. Add the chicken and noodles to the vegetables, pour over the sauce, and heat through.

Mulligatawny Chicken

This recipe has a tomato base and a mild curry flavor which children love. It has been a family favorite since I was a child and was invented by my mother. It is best served with rice and, for special occasions, you can serve *poppadums* as an accompaniment. They are available in most grocery stores.

MAKES 8 ADULT PORTIONS

1 chicken, cut into about 10 pieces, skinned
seasoned flour
vegetable oil
2 medium onions, peeled and chopped
6 tablespoons tomato paste
2 tablespoons mild curry powder
3³/₄ cups chicken broth (see page 62)

1 large or 2 small dessert apples, cored and thinly sliced
1 small carrot, peeled and thinly sliced
2 lemon slices
¹/₂ cup golden raisins
1 bay leaf
2 teaspoons brown sugar

Coat the chicken pieces with seasoned flour. Fry in vegetable oil until golden brown. Drain on paper towels and place in a Dutch oven.

Fry the onions in a little oil until golden, then stir in the tomato paste. Add the curry powder and continue stirring for 2 minutes over a low heat. Stir in 2 tablespoons flour, then pour in 1¹/₄ cups of the broth, mixing well.

Add the apples, carrot, lemon slices, golden raisins, bay leaf, and the rest of the broth. Season with brown sugar, salt, and pepper. Pour the sauce over the chicken in the Dutch oven, cover, and cook for 1 hour in an oven preheated to 350°F. Remove the lemon slices and bay leaf; take the chicken off the bone and cut it into pieces.

Sesame Chicken Nuggets with Chinese Sauce

These crisp sesame-coated nuggets are very popular. They are good served with Special Fried Rice (see page 123). It's fun for children to eat these with chopsticks – you can buy plastic ones that are joined at the top and are very easy for children to use. Sesame seeds can cause an allergic reaction in young children. Although this is very rare, watch your child closely, particularly if he is allergic to any other foods, or has any conditions such as eczema or asthma.

MAKES 12 NUGGETS

1 double chicken breast, off the bone
and skinned
1 egg
1 tablespoon milk
a little salt and pepper
all-purpose flour
sesame seeds for coating
2 tablespoons vegetable oil

Chinese Sauce
1 cup chicken broth (see page 62)
2 teaspoons soy sauce
1 teaspoon sesame oil
1 tablespoon sugar
1 teaspoon cider vinegar
1 tablespoon cornstarch
1 scallion, finely sliced

Cut each half of the chicken breast into about 6 pieces. Beat the egg and milk together. Dip the nuggets into the seasoned flour, then into the egg mixture and finally coat with the sesame seeds. Fry in hot oil for about 5 minutes, turning the chicken frequently, until golden brown and cooked through. Drain on paper towels and keep warm. Meanwhile, mix together all the ingredients for the sauce (except the scallion) in a small saucepan. Bring to a boil, then simmer for 2–3 minutes or until thickened. Add the scallion and pour the sauce over the chicken nuggets.

Marinated Chicken on the Griddle

I love cooking chicken, meat, or fish on a griddle, and it's a very healthy way of cooking as it uses very little fat. My three children love this recipe as marinating the chicken gives it a lovely flavor and makes it more tender. Make sure the griddle is really hot before you lay the food on it.

MAKES 2 ADULT PORTIONS

2 chicken breasts
1 tablespoon olive oil

1 tablespoon soy sauce
1 tablespoon honey
1 small garlic clove, peeled and sliced
2 sprigs of fresh rosemary (optional)

Marinade
juice of ½ lemon

Score the chicken breasts 2 or 3 times with a sharp knife. Mix together all the ingredients for the marinade and marinate the chicken for at least 2 hours. Heat the griddle, brush with oil, then remove the chicken from the marinade and cook for 4–5 minutes on each side or until cooked through. Cut into strips and serve with French fries or mashed potato, and colorful vegetables such as carrots, broccoli, or peas.

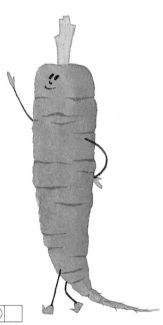

MEAT

Annabel's Juicy Burgers

The grated apple makes these burgers really moist. Serve in a hamburger bun with salad and tomato catsup, and some oven-baked French fries. They are also good cooked over hot coals on a barbecue.

MAKES 8 BURGERS

½ red bell pepper, seeded and chopped
1 onion, peeled and finely chopped
1 tablespoon vegetable oil
2 cups lean ground beef or lamb
1 tablespoon fresh parsley, chopped
1 chicken bouillon cube, finely crumbled
1 apple, peeled and grated

1 egg, lightly beaten
½ cup fresh bread crumbs
1 teaspoon Worcestershire sauce
salt and freshly ground black pepper
a little all-purpose flour
vegetable oil for brushing a griddle pan
or for frying

Fry the red bell pepper and half the onion in the vegetable oil for about 5 minutes or until softened. In a mixing bowl, combine the sautéed onion, bell pepper, and remaining raw onion with all the ingredients except the flour and vegetable oil. With floured hands, form into 8 burgers. Brush a griddle pan with a little oil and, when hot, place 4 burgers on the griddle and cook for about 5 minutes each side or until browned and cooked through. Repeat with the remaining burgers. Alternately, fry in a little hot oil in a shallow skillet. Serve the burgers on their own or in a toasted hamburger bun with salad and catsup.

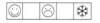

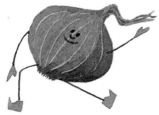

Cocktail Meatballs with Tomato Sauce

These meatballs can be served on their own without the sauce and make tasty finger food. They are also good served with spaghetti or rice.

MAKES 6 PORTIONS

Tomato Sauce
1½ tablespoons light olive oil
1 medium onion, peeled and chopped
1 garlic clove, crushed
9 oz fresh ripe tomatoes, skinned, seeded, and chopped
14 oz canned chopped tomatoes
1 teaspoon balsamic vinegar
1 teaspoon superfine sugar
salt and freshly ground black pepper
1 tablespoon fresh basil, torn

Meatballs
2 cups lean ground beef
1 onion, peeled and finely chopped
1 dessert apple, peeled and grated
1 cup fresh white bread crumbs
1 tablespoon fresh parsley, chopped
1 chicken bouillon cube, crumbled and dissolved in 2 tablespoons boiling water
salt and freshly ground black pepper
all-purpose flour for forming meatballs
vegetable oil for frying

To make the tomato sauce, heat the oil in a saucepan and gently cook the onion and garlic until softened. Stir in the fresh tomatoes and cook for 1 minute. Add the canned tomatoes, balsamic vinegar, sugar, and seasoning and cook for 20 minutes over a low heat. Add the basil and then blend in a food processor to make a smooth sauce.

Meanwhile, mix together the ingredients for the meatballs. Using floured hands, form into about 24 balls. Heat the oil in a skillet and sauté the meatballs over a fairly high heat, turning occasionally, until browned, then reduce the heat and continue to cook for about 5 minutes. Pour over the tomato sauce and continue to cook, covered, for about 10–15 minutes.

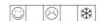

Shepherd's Pie

This is traditional British winter fare. It is very nice to make your child his very own little shepherd's pie. Let him see it and then spoon out of the hot dish on to his plate.

MAKES 4 ADULT PORTIONS

1 onion, peeled and finely chopped
1 small red bell pepper, seeded and
finely chopped
1 tablespoon parsley, finely chopped
2 tablespoons vegetable oil
2 cups lean ground beef
1 cup chicken broth (see page 62) or
beef broth
1 tablespoon tomato catsup
1/2 tablespoon Worcestershire sauce

salt and pepper
1 1/2 cups mushrooms, washed and sliced
1 tablespoon butter or margarine

Topping
4 cups potato, peeled and chopped
1 1/2 tablespoons butter
1/4 cup milk
salt and pepper

Fry the chopped onion, bell pepper, and parsley in the oil until softened. Meanwhile, in a skillet, brown the ground meat. Chop the meat in a food processor for 30 seconds to make it easier to chew. Stir into the onion mixture and add the broth, catsup, Worcestershire sauce, and seasoning. Cook over a low heat for about 20 minutes. Meanwhile, sauté the mushrooms in the butter or margarine and add these to the meat when it is cooked.

To make the topping, boil the potato in lightly salted water for about 15 minutes or until tender. Mash them together with half the butter, the milk, and some salt and pepper. Spread over the meat either in one large dish or in four individual dishes, then cook in an oven preheated to 350°F for 10 minutes. Dot the top with the remaining butter and put under a hot broiler for about 3 minutes or until golden.

Mini Minute Steaks

These mini steaks, with a delicious gravy and sautéed potatoes, are absolutely wonderful.

MAKES 2 ADULT OR 4 CHILD PORTIONS

2 tablespoons vegetable oil
1 onion, peeled and thinly sliced
1 teaspoon superfine sugar
1 tablespoon water
⅞ cup beef broth
1 teaspoon cornstarch mixed with
1 tablespoon water

a few drops of Worcestershire sauce
1 teaspoon tomato paste
salt and pepper
3 cups potato, peeled
1½ tablespoons butter
2½ oz minute steaks (fillet or rump),
about ¼ inch thick

To make the gravy, heat 1 tablespoon of the vegetable oil in a skillet. Add the onion and cook for 7–8 minutes until just turning golden brown. Stir in the sugar and water, increase the heat and cook for about 1 minute until the water has evaporated. Stir in the beef broth, cornstarch mixed with water, Worcestershire sauce, and tomato paste. Season with salt and pepper. Cook, stirring, for 2–3 minutes until thickened.

For the sautéed potato, cut the potato into large chunks, bring to a boil in lightly salted water, and cook for about 8 minutes until they are just tender. Drain and cut into ½-inch thick slices. Heat the butter in a skillet and sauté the potato for 5–6 minutes, turning occasionally until golden brown and crispy.

Heat the remaining oil in a skillet, season the steaks, and fry for 1–2 minutes each side. Serve with the gravy and sautéed potato.

Veal Stroganoff

Veal is easier than beef for your toddler to chew. This recipe is quick and easy to make and delicious. It is very nice as a family meal served with noodles and, to give it an authentic stroganoff taste, you can even add a spoonful of sour cream.

MAKES 2 ADULT PORTIONS

vegetable oil for sautéing
1 onion, peeled and finely chopped
½ red and ½ yellow bell pepper, seeded and cut into strips
8 oz thin veal scallop, cut into strips

all-purpose flour
salt and pepper
1¼ cups chicken broth (see page 62)
2 cups mushrooms, washed and sliced

Heat a little oil in a skillet and sauté the onion for 3–4 minutes. Add the strips of bell pepper and continue to cook for 1 more minute. Roll the strips of veal in seasoned flour and cook these in the skillet for about 3 minutes or until browned (add a little more oil if you find the veal is sticking to the pan).

Pour the chicken broth over the veal. Stir in the mushrooms and salt and pepper to taste. Simmer, covered, for 8 minutes.

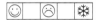

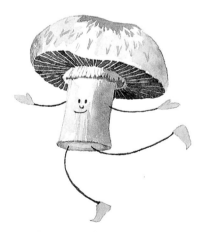

Sticky Chops

MAKES 2 ADULT PORTIONS

Marinade
2 tablespoons tomato catsup
1 tablespoon soy sauce
1 tablespoon runny honey
1 teaspoon lemon juice

a few drops of Worcestershire sauce
a little freshly ground black pepper

4 lamb chops or lamb cutlets

Mix together all of the ingredients for the marinade, add the lamb chops, and leave to marinate for 1–2 hours at room temperature or overnight in the refrigerator. Place on a broiler pan under a medium-high broiler for 4–5 minutes each side, basting with any remaining marinade.

Liver and Onion

MAKES 1–2 ADULT PORTIONS

½ onion, peeled and chopped
1 tablespoon green bell pepper,
finely chopped
vegetable oil

2 tablespoons mushrooms, chopped
1 medium tomato, skinned, seeded,
and chopped
4 oz calf's liver

Fry the chopped onion and bell pepper in a little oil until the onion is very brown. Add the chopped mushrooms and tomato and fry for another 2 minutes. Fry the liver for 1½ minutes each side. When the liver is cooked, cut into small pieces and cover with the vegetables.

PASTA

Spaghetti with Two-Tomato Sauce

A really good home-made tomato sauce is always popular – and it can be served with any type of pasta and maybe freshly grated Parmesan cheese.

MAKES 4 CHILD PORTIONS

3 tablespoons olive oil
1 onion, peeled and chopped
1 garlic clove, peeled and crushed
4 ripe tomatoes, skinned, seeded
and chopped
14 oz canned chopped tomatoes

pinch of sugar
1 bay leaf
2 tablespoons fresh basil, chopped
salt and pepper
9 oz spaghetti

Heat the oil in a saucepan and sauté the onion and garlic for 5–6 minutes until softened. Add the fresh and canned tomatoes, sugar, bay leaf, and basil, then season with salt and pepper. Bring to a simmer and cook for 20 minutes. Meanwhile, cook the spaghetti according to the packet instructions. Drain the pasta and mix with the sauce.

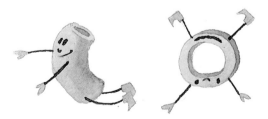

Bow-Ties with Swiss Cheese and Cherry Tomatoes

This is a great favorite with my children and can be eaten either warm or cold.

MAKES 4 CHILD PORTIONS

1³⁄₄ cups bow-tie pasta
1 tablespoon white wine vinegar
3 tablespoons olive oil
½ teaspoon Dijon mustard (optional)
a pinch of sugar

a little salt and freshly ground black pepper
1 tablespoon fresh chives, snipped
4 oz cherry tomatoes, halved or quartered
½ cup Swiss cheese, grated

Cook the pasta in lightly salted water according to the packet instructions. Make a vinaigrette by mixing together the vinegar, oil, mustard (if using), sugar, and seasoning, then add the snipped chives. Drain the pasta and put into a bowl, then mix with the cherry tomatoes and Swiss cheese. Shake the vinaigrette, pour over the pasta, and toss well to coat.

Fluffy Macaroni and Cheese

Whipped egg whites give this tasty macaroni and cheese dish a lovely light texture.

MAKES 4 PORTIONS

3 cups macaroni
1½ tablespoons butter
¼ cup flour
1¼ cups milk
a little nutmeg, grated
¼ cup mascarpone cheese

½ cup Cheddar cheese, grated
¼ cup Swiss cheese, grated
2 eggs, separated
salt and freshly ground black pepper
4 tablespoons Parmesan cheese, freshly grated

Cook the macaroni according to the packet instructions. Use the butter, flour, milk, and nutmeg to make a thick white sauce (see page 59). Remove from the heat and whisk in the Cheddar and Swiss cheese until melted, and then the mascarpone and egg yolks. Season with salt and pepper.

Whisk the egg whites to form soft peaks and gently fold into the sauce. Drain the pasta, mix with the sauce, and spoon into an ovenproof dish. Sprinkle the Parmesan on top and place in an oven preheated to 350°F for 12–15 minutes until lightly golden.

Spaghetti Primavera

A simple recipe for spaghetti with spring vegetables in a tasty cheese sauce. You could also make this with pasta shapes.

MAKES 4 PORTIONS

5 oz spaghetti
1 tablespoon olive oil
1 onion, chopped
1 garlic clove, crushed
1 medium carrot (approx. 3 oz) cut into matchsticks
1 medium zucchini (approx. 3 oz) cut into matchsticks

1 good cup cauliflower cut into small florets
¾ cup light crème fraîche
¾ cup vegetable broth (see page 33)
½ cup frozen peas
½ cup fresh Parmesan cheese, grated

Cook the spaghetti according to the packet instructions. Heat the oil in a heavy-based saucepan and sauté the onion and garlic for 1 minute. Add the carrot and zucchini matchsticks and sauté, stirring occasionally, for 2–3 minutes. Meanwhile, blanch the cauliflower in lightly salted boiling water for 5 minutes or steam until tender. Add the crème fraîche, vegetable broth, and peas to the carrot and zucchini and stir in. Cook for 2–3 minutes before stirring in the Parmesan. Drain the spaghetti and toss with the sauce.

Bow-Ties with Tomato and Mozzarella Sauce

A very tasty, easy-to-prepare tomato sauce enriched with two cheeses.

MAKES 4 CHILD PORTIONS

1½ cups bow-tie pasta
2 tablespoons olive oil
1 onion, peeled and chopped
1 garlic clove, peeled and crushed
14 oz canned chopped tomatoes
1 teaspoon balsamic vinegar
a pinch of sugar

1 tablespoon fresh basil, torn
a scant ½ cup vegetable broth (see page 33)
1⅛ cups mozzarella cheese, diced
3 tablespoons Parmesan cheese, grated
salt and pepper

Cook the pasta according to the packet instructions. To make the sauce, heat the olive oil in a saucepan and sauté the onion and garlic for 5–6 minutes until softened. Stir in the chopped tomatoes, balsamic vinegar, sugar, basil, and broth, and simmer for 10 minutes. Stir in the mozzarella and Parmesan cheeses. Season to taste and mix with the bow-tie pasta.

Animal Pasta Salad with Multicolored Vegetables

I make this recipe with multicolored, animal-shaped pasta. Toddlers love picking out all the different ingredients. It looks very attractive and colorful on a plate and can be served warm or cold.
You can omit the chicken for a vegetarian dish.

MAKES 4 ADULT PORTIONS

1 1/8 cups multicolored pasta shapes
1 single chicken breast, skinned and cut
into bite-sized pieces
vegetable oil
3 baby carrots, or 1 medium carrot, cut
into fine strips
1/2 cup each of cauliflower and broccoli
florets
3 zucchini, trimmed and sliced
1/2 cup green beans, chopped
2/3 cup frozen corn kernels

1/2 red bell pepper, finely chopped
salt
sugar

Dressing
2 tablespoons cider vinegar
1/2 teaspoon salt and a little black
pepper
1/4 cup olive oil
2 scallions, finely sliced, or
2 tablespoons snipped chives

Cook the pasta according to the packet instructions and drain. Fry the chicken in a little oil for 2 minutes, then add the carrots and continue to cook for a further 5 minutes. Meanwhile, steam the cauliflower, broccoli, zucchini, and beans until cooked but still crisp. The cauliflower and broccoli will need a little longer than the zucchini and beans. Cook the corn and red bell pepper in water with a little salt and sugar for 5 minutes.

To prepare the dressing, whisk the vinegar with the salt and pepper, then whisk in the olive oil, a little at a time. Add the scallions or chives. Combine all the ingredients together and pour over the dressing.

FRUIT AND DESSERTS

Poached Fruits

MAKES 4 ADULT PORTIONS

*2 large or 3 small pears, peeled,
quartered, and cored
5 oz plums, halved and pitted
1 good cup blackberries*

*⅜ cup apple juice
⅓ cup superfine sugar
1 small stick cinnamon
¾ cup raspberries*

Cut the pear quarters in half and place in a large saucepan. Add the plums, blackberries, apple juice, superfine sugar, and cinnamon stick. Bring to a gentle simmer and cover for 10 minutes. Stir in the raspberries. Remove the cinnamon stick before serving and serve chilled.

Peach Melba Delight

A healthy alternate to this favorite ice-cream dessert.

MAKES 1 ADULT PORTION

*¾ cup raspberries
2 teaspoons superfine sugar
⅝ cup plain yogurt*

*1 ripe peach, skinned, pitted, and cut
into small pieces*

Put the raspberries and sugar in a small saucepan and cook gently for 2–3 minutes or until soft. Press the raspberries through a strainer and mix together with the yogurt and peach.

Snow-Covered Fruit Salad

Try this combination of fruits, which are all rich in vitamin C – better than any vitamin tablets. You can make your own combination according to what is in season. If you have a melon scooper, scoop the melon into small balls.

MAKES 5 ADULT PORTIONS

1 peach, skinned, pitted, and cut into small pieces
1 papaya, peeled, seeded, and cut into small chunks
8 strawberries, washed, hulled, and cut into quarters
2 oranges, peeled, white skin removed, and cut into chunks
1 tablespoon blueberries or raspberries
½ small cantaloupe melon, flesh removed and cut into chunks

1 cup cherries, pitted and halved
1 small wedge of watermelon, flesh removed and cut into chunks
2 kiwi fruit, peeled and sliced
juice of 1 orange

Topping
2 cups plain yogurt
2 tablespoons honey
2 tablespoons wheatgerm or muesli (optional)

Combine all the fruits together in a large bowl. Pour the orange juice over them and mix well.

Mix the yogurt with the honey and wheatgerm or muesli, if using, and pour over the fruit just before serving.

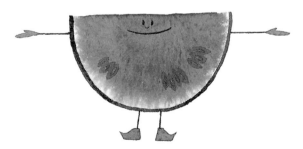

Peaches with Amaretti Biscuits

Amaretti biscuits are small, round macaroons from Italy, and can be bought in most grocery stores. This delicious fruit dessert can be made with many different fruits. Try a combination of white peaches and raspberries or sliced plums. You could also make this dessert using light crème fraîche.

MAKES 2 ADULT PORTIONS

2 large, ripe peaches, pitted and sliced
1 oz amaretti biscuits, crushed

a scant ⅝ cup crème fraîche
1 heaped tablespoon brown sugar

Place the sliced peaches in a shallow ovenproof dish and sprinkle with the crushed amaretti biscuits. Cover with the crème fraîche and then sprinkle over the brown sugar. Place under a preheated broiler for about 6 minutes until golden.

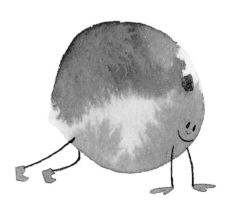

Pear, Apple, and Raspberry Crumble

A delicious crumble bursting with fruit is comfort food at its very best. It's easy to prepare and always a great favorite with my family. I like to choose fruits that have a slightly tart flavor. Rhubarb with $1/4$ cup brown sugar and a little orange juice makes a good fruit crumble, and the apple and blackberry mixture on page 86 mixed with $1/2$ cup soft brown sugar is also delicious. Crumbles are best served hot with custard sauce or vanilla ice cream.

MAKES 6 ADULT PORTIONS

*2 dessert apples, peeled, cored,
and chopped
2 ripe pears, peeled, cored, and chopped
2 cups raspberries, fresh or frozen
1 tablespoon superfine sugar*

Crumble Topping
*$1^{1}/_{4}$ cups all-purpose flour
a pinch of salt
$1/2$ cup cold butter, cut into pieces
$3/8$ cup soft brown sugar
$2/3$ cup oatmeal*

To make the crumble topping, mix together the flour and salt and cut in the butter until the mixture resembles bread crumbs. Stir in the sugar and oatmeal.

Mix together the apples, pears, and raspberries in a suitable ovenproof dish (I use a 10 x 8 inch oval dish), sprinkle over the sugar, and top with the crumble mixture. Bake in an oven preheated to 350°F for 30 minutes, by which time the top of the crumble should have turned a golden brown.

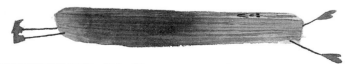

American-Style Cheesecake

This is one of the most delicious cheesecakes I have ever tasted. Serve it plain or with the cherry topping.

MAKES 10 ADULT PORTIONS

Base
9 oz graham crackers
a good ½ cup butter

Filling
1 cup superfine sugar
3 tablespoons cornstarch
3 cups cream cheese
2 eggs

1 teaspoon vanilla extract or grated zest
of ½ lemon
1¼ cups whipping cream
½ cup golden raisins (optional)

Topping
15 oz canned cherries in syrup
½ tablespoon cornstarch

To make the base, break the cookies into pieces, put them in a plastic bag, and crush them with a rolling pin. Melt the butter and stir in the crushed cookies. Line a 9-inch springform cake pan with baking paper and grease the sides. Press the crushed-cookie mixture over the base.

For the filling, mix the sugar and cornstarch. Beat in the cream cheese. Add the eggs and vanilla (or lemon zest). Beat until smooth. Slowly whisk in the cream until thickened. Stir in the golden raisins. Pour over the cookie base. Bake for 1 hour in an oven pre-heated to 350°F. Cool.

For the topping, drain the cherries, reserving ½ cup syrup. Mix the cornstarch with 1 tablespoon of the syrup. Pour the remaining syrup into a saucepan, stir in the cornstarch mixture, and bring to a boil, stirring until thick. Cool. Decorate the cheesecake with circles of cherries and pour over the glaze.

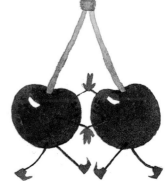

Fruit Suckers

Suckers are always popular with children. You can buy molds with reusable plastic sticks. Fill the molds with your chosen fruit purée, juice, or smoothie, put the plastic sticks on top (these also serve as covers), and freeze on a level surface in the freezer. Dip the molds into warm water when you want to get the suckers out.

You can make your own fruit purées from fresh fruits in season, or you can use use natural fruit juices. Experiment with different combinations such as nectarine, strawberry, and orange juice. Sweeten to taste (if wished) with sugar or honey, and stir in plain or fruit-flavored yogurt for a frozen yogurt sucker. These pure ingredients are much better for your child than commercial iced suckers, many of which are full of additives, colorings, and sugar.

My son Nicholas, at two years old, had quite sophisticated taste and developed a liking for passion-fruit suckers. Try also pineapple juice, concentrated orange juice, and sparkling apple juice. Two-tone suckers are fun. Half-fill the molds with fruit purée or juice of one color, freeze, then pour over a purée or juice of a contrasting color.

Peach and Passion-Fruit Suckers

MAKES 6 SUCKERS

*2 large oranges, squeezed
strained juice of 3 passion fruit*

*2 juicy, ripe peaches, skinned, pitted,
and chopped*

Combine all the ingredients in a blender or food processor and blend until smooth. Pour into the sucker molds and freeze.

Cranberry, Lemonade, and Orange Suckers

A great-tasting combination, these suckers take only minutes to prepare.

MAKES 4 LARGE OR 6 SMALL SUCKERS

1 cup cranberry juice
½ cup lemonade

½ cup fresh orange juice

Combine all the ingredients together and pour into molds.

Grandma's Lokshen Pudding

Lokshen is vermicelli: very fine egg noodles. This easy dessert is one of my all-time favorites. For variation, add a few slivered almonds.

MAKES 4 ADULT PORTIONS

3 cups vermicelli
1 large egg, beaten
2 tablespoons butter, melted
1 cup milk

1 tablespoon vanilla sugar or superfine sugar
½ teaspoon apple pie spice
½ cup each golden raisins and raisins

Cook the vermicelli in boiling water for about 5 minutes. Drain and mix with the remaining ingredients. Place in a greased, shallow baking dish, and bake in an oven preheated to 350°F for about 30 minutes.

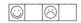

Frozen Strawberry-Yogurt Ice Cream

A delicious easy-to-make frozen-yogurt ice cream using only natural ingredients. You can also make a peach melba frozen yogurt using fresh raspberries, puréed and strained, and peach yogurt. I like to serve this in a tall glass with fresh berries.

MAKES 6 ADULT PORTIONS

½ cup superfine sugar
1¼ cups water
3 cups fresh strawberries

1¼ cups strawberry yogurt
⅝ cup heavy cream, whipped
1 egg white, beaten

Put the sugar in a saucepan with the water. Bring to a boil and continue to boil for 5 minutes to make a syrup. Set aside to cool for a few minutes. Purée the strawberries and press through a strainer, then mix with the syrup and stir in the strawberry yogurt and whipped cream. Churn for 10 minutes in an ice-cream-making machine, then fold in the beaten egg white, and churn for another 10 minutes or until firm.

This can also be made without an ice-cream-making machine but it will be more time-consuming. Pour the mixture into a plastic container and freeze. Remove and whisk when semi-frozen, then return to the freezer. Whisk again after 1 hour. Fold in the whipped egg white, freeze again, and whisk two more times during the freezing process.

BAKING FOR TODDLERS

Funny-Shape Cookies

Cookie cutters come in all sorts of weird and wonderful shapes. I use a gingerbread cutter and animal cutouts and my son can't wait to get his hands on the cookies. I get a running commentary as to which piece of the anatomy he has just eaten!

MAKES 15–20 COOKIES (DEPENDING ON SIZE OF CUTTERS)

1/2 cup wholewheat flour
1 cup all-purpose flour
1/2 cup semolina
1/4 teaspoon each ground ginger, cinnamon, and salt

3/8 cup margarine or butter
1 medium, ripe banana
1 1/2 tablespoons maple syrup
cream cheese, for spreading
a few raisins

Put the flours, semolina, ginger, cinnamon, and salt in a mixing bowl and cut in the margarine or butter. Mash the banana well with the maple syrup and stir into the mixture to make a smooth, pliable dough.

Roll out on a lightly floured surface and cut into shapes with cookie cutters. Bake on lightly greased cookie sheets in an oven preheated to 400°F for 20 minutes until golden and firm. Cool on a wire rack. If you wish, spread the cooled cookies with cream cheese, marking with a fork to represent the various animals' fur. Use pieces of raisin for eyes and noses.

Apple Flowers

You can use ready-rolled sheets of puff pastry, which only need to be unrolled and baked – so it couldn't be simpler to make these delicious pastries. Alternately, use a block of puff pastry and roll it out yourself.

MAKES 6 MINI APPLE TARTS

11 oz puff pastry
2 tablespoons butter
a scant ¼ cup superfine sugar
1 egg
a few drops of almond extract
½ cup ground almonds

1½ tablespoons melted butter
3 small dessert apples
superfine sugar for sprinkling
2 tablespoons apricot jelly, strained
1 tablespoon lemon juice
6 candied cherries

Preheat the oven to 400°F. Cut 6 circles out of the pastry using a round pastry cutter (approx. 4 inches) or cut around a plate using a sharp knife. To make the almond filling, cream together the butter and sugar until soft, then beat in the egg, a few drops of almond extract, and the ground almonds, to make a smooth cream. Prick the pastry a few times with a fork and brush with a little melted butter. Spread some of the almond cream over each of the circles.

Peel and core the apples, then cut in half and slice thinly. Arrange the sliced fruit around the pastry circles. Brush with a little melted butter, sprinkle over some superfine sugar, and bake in the oven for about 20 minutes or until the pastry is crisp and the fruit is cooked. Transfer the tarts to a wire rack to cool.

Warm the jelly and lemon juice in a small saucepan and then brush the fruit with a little of the melted, strained, apricot jelly to glaze the tarts. Decorate the center of each tart with a candied cherry.

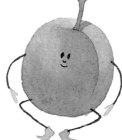

Candy Cup Cakes

These little cakes can be frozen, which is best done before they are frosted. They are ideal for a birthday celebration, and it's fun to decorate them with faces using candy and tubes of writing frosting.

MAKES 12 CAKES

1/2 cup sweet butter or soft margarine
1/2 cup superfine sugar
2 eggs
1 1/4 cups self-rising flour
1 teaspoon vanilla extract

Cream Cheese Frosting
1/4 cup sweet butter
2 cups powdered sugar, sifted
1 teaspoon vanilla extract
1/2 cup cream cheese

Colored Frosting
2 cups powdered sugar, sifted
about 2 tablespoons water
a few drops of food coloring

Decoration
1 packet candy-coated chocolate beans
1 packet colored candy shapes
assorted colors of writing frosting
in tubes

Chocolate Frosting
1/4 cup sweet butter
3/4 cup powdered sugar, sifted
1 tablespoon cocoa powder

Cream the butter or margarine and sugar together until light and fluffy, then beat in the eggs, one at a time with 1 tablespoon of flour. Add the vanilla and fold in the remaining flour. Half-fill 12 little paper cups set into cup-cake pans and bake in an oven preheated to 350°F for 15–20 minutes. Remove and cool on a wire rack.

I like to make 2 different colored frostings, so I use chocolate and then a pale cream cheese frosting. If you prefer, make a simple colored frosting. Mix the powdered sugar with enough water to form a spreading consistency, divide into two, and stir in the coloring of your choice.

For the chocolate frosting, cut the butter into small pieces and beat with a wooden spoon until creamy. Beat in the sugar, a little at a time, then beat in the cocoa powder.

For the cream cheese frosting, beat the butter, sugar, and vanilla until crumbly. Stir in the cream cheese. Do not overbeat or it will become watery. Spread over the cakes. Decorate them with funny faces made with candy-coated chocolate beans, colored candy, and writing frosting.

Pineapple and Raisin Muffins

These are absolutely delicious, and very healthy, too; they never last long in our house!

MAKES ABOUT 13 MUFFINS

1 cup all-purpose flour
1 cup wholewheat flour
1 teaspoon baking powder
³/₄ teaspoon baking soda
1 teaspoon powdered cinnamon
1 teaspoon powdered ginger
¹/₂ teaspoon salt

³/₄ cup vegetable oil
³/₈ cup superfine sugar
2 eggs
1¹/₈ cups carrot, grated
8 oz crushed pineapple, drained
²/₃ cup raisins

Sift together the flours, baking powder, baking soda, cinnamon, ginger, and salt and mix well. Beat the oil, sugar, and eggs together until well blended. Add the grated carrot, pineapple, and raisins. Gradually add the flour mixture, beating just enough to combine all the ingredients. Pour the batter into muffin cups and bake in an oven preheated to 350°F for about 25 minutes or until well risen and golden. Cool on a wire rack.

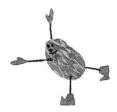

Yogurt Processor Cake

This cake has a lovely flavor and a very moist texture. It takes no more than five minutes to prepare. You can also make it in two round cake pans. Beat 1 cup whipping cream with 2 tablespoons superfine sugar and fold in ³/₄ cup raspberries. Use to sandwich the two cakes together.

MAKES 8 ADULT PORTIONS

a scant ³/₄ cup superfine sugar
1 cup vegetable oil
1 cup plain set yogurt
2 eggs

2 cups all-purpose flour
3 teaspoons baking powder
2 teaspoons vanilla extract
powdered sugar

Grease a 10-inch, round tube pan. In a blender or food processor, mix the sugar with the oil, then add the yogurt and mix. Blend with the eggs, flour, baking powder, and vanilla. Pour into the prepared pan and bake at 325°F for about 50 minutes. Sift sugar over the top when cold.

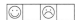

White-Chocolate-Button Cookies

These are so easy to make and are really delicious. Baked for only 12 minutes, they should be quite soft when they are taken out of the oven so that when they cool down they are really moist.

MAKES 20 COOKIES

¹/₂ cup sweet butter or margarine at
room temperature
¹/₂ cup superfine sugar
¹/₂ cup brown sugar
1 egg
1 teaspoon vanilla extract

1¹/₂ cups all-purpose flour
¹/₂ teaspoon baking powder
¹/₄ teaspoon salt
1 cup white-chocolate buttons
¹/₂ cup pecans or walnuts, chopped
(optional)

Beat the butter or margarine together with the sugars. Beat the egg and vanilla together with a fork, then beat them into the butter mixture. In a bowl, mix together the flour, baking powder, and salt. Add this to the butter and egg, and blend well.

Break the chocolate buttons into pieces with a rolling pin, or in a food processor, and stir, with the nuts (if using), into the batter.

Line several cookie sheets with nonstick baking paper and roll the batter into walnut-sized balls. Put these on to the sheets, spaced well apart, and bake in an oven preheated to 375°F for 12 minutes. Carefully lift the cookies off the baking paper and let cool.

My Favorite Chocolate Cookie Squares

These are great for a children's party or supper-time treat.

MAKES 16 CHOCOLATE COOKIE SQUARES

4 oz graham crackers
4 oz ginger snaps
5 oz milk chocolate
4 oz plain chocolate
⅓ cup light molasses or light corn syrup

⅜ cup unsalted butter
¾ cup ready-to-eat dried apricots, chopped
⅓ cup raisins
1½ oz Rice Krispies

Lightly grease and line an 8-inch, square, shallow tin. Put the graham crackers in a plastic bag and crush with a rolling pin to form coarse crumbs. Melt the chocolate, molasses or syrup, and butter in a heatproof bowl over a pan of simmering water. Stir in the graham cracker crumbs until well coated, then add the apricots and raisins and, finally, stir in the Rice Krispies.

Spoon the mixture into the tin. Level the surface, pressing down with a masher, and put in the refrigerator to set. Cut into squares before serving.

Thumbprint Jelly Cookies

So called because you stick your thumb in the middle of the dough
to make a hollow for the jelly. The deeper you stick your thumb,
the more jelly you get. Use your child's favorite jelly or make
different flavored jelly cookies.

MAKES 25 SMALL COOKIES

¹/₂ cup butter
¹/₄ cup superfine sugar
1 egg yolk
¹/₂ teaspoon almond extract

1¹/₂ cups all-purpose flour
pinch of salt
strawberry jelly or a selection of
different jellies

Beat the butter with the sugar, then blend in the egg yolk and almond
extract. Gradually add the flour and salt and mix to a dough. Take
walnut-sized pieces of dough, flatten slightly, and press your thumb in the
center to leave an indentation. Place on a cookie sheet lined with nonstick
baking paper. Fill the indentations with half a teaspoon of jelly and bake
in an oven preheated to 350°F for 10 minutes.

Cheese Pretzels

These are delicious and great fun to make. Your children will enjoy helping you twist the pretzels into different shapes. You can even make letters of the alphabet and spell your child's name!

MAKES 20 PRETZELS

3 teaspoons dried yeast
1 cup warm water
3 cups all-purpose flour
½ teaspoon salt

1¼ cups Cheddar cheese, grated
2 tablespoons vegetable oil
1 tablespoon sea salt
1 tablespoon sesame seeds

Dissolve the yeast in the warm water. Sift the flour and salt into a large bowl and stir in the cheese, oil, and yeast liquid. Bring together to form a dough and knead on a floured surface for 10 minutes by hand, or for 5 minutes using a dough hook. Place in an oiled bowl, cover with saran wrap, and leave in a warm place for about 1 hour. Break off small pieces of dough, roll into 10-inch-long strands and twist into pretzel shapes. Arrange on a greased cookie sheet. Brush with oil and sprinkle some with sea salt and some with sesame seeds. Bake in an oven preheated to 400°F for 15 minutes until golden brown.

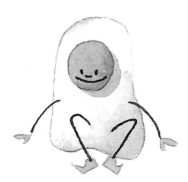

HEALTHY SNACKS

Fruit Snacks

Wash fruit well. Peel, core, seed,
or pit and trim as needed.

Bananas, whole or cut into pieces

Chunks of peeled and cored
apples

Chunks of pear, cored

Orange, mandarin, or tangerine
segments with as much of the
white skin removed as possible
(make sure there are no seeds)

Kiwi fruit, peeled and sliced

Strawberries, hulled and halved

Seedless grapes, skinned for
babies under one year

Melon, peeled, seeded, and cut
into bite-sized pieces

Peaches, skinned, pitted, and
sliced

Mango, peeled, pitted, and sliced

Papaya, peeled, seeds removed,
and cut in thick slices

Raspberries, washed carefully

Litchis, peeled and pitted (toddlers
can easily choke on litchi pits)

Pineapple, peeled and cut into
chunks

Dried fruit, such as apricots,
prunes and raisins (if too tough,
soak in boiling water).

Chocolate-Dipped Fruit

A very appealing way of giving
fruit to children is to melt some
dark chocolate in a double boiler,
dip the tip of the fruit piece into
the chocolate, and pierce the fruit
with a toothpick. Stick the toothpicks with the fruit into an orange
and put this into the refrigerator to
allow the chocolate to harden.
Strawberries, pineapple chunks,
and orange or tangerine segments
are especially nice. Remember to
remove the toothpicks before giving the fruit to your child.

Whole bananas can be coated
in chocolate. Place on waxed
paper and freeze or chill until the
chocolate has set.

If you are worried about your
child having too much chocolate,
use carob as a substitute.

SNACKS THAT WON'T HARM YOUR CHILD'S TEETH

Vegetable Snacks

As with fruit, wash, peel, trim, and seed as appropriate.

Toddlers love to dip raw vegetables into a sauce, and an attractively arranged selection of crudités is great for a toddler who is teething. You can buy packs of peeled mini carrots in the grocery store, and these are ideal for toddlers, as are strips of red bell pepper, sugar snap peas, sticks of cucumber, and cherry tomatoes. Try giving your child some simple but delicious dips like the Green Goddess Dip (see page 182), or make one by combining sour cream or cream cheese, a little catsup, some chives, and seasoning. You can also buy ready-made dips such as *hummus* – made from garbanzo beans – which is very nutritious.

Carrots and white cabbage, grated and mixed with a little mayonnaise and raisins, make a simple and nutritious snack piled onto lettuce leaves.

Cheese Snacks

Cheese makes an ideal snack for toddlers. Try using a cookie cutter to make animal shapes from slices of cheese. Edam, Monterey Jack, and Swiss are particular favorites with most children. Individual cheeses like the small, round Babybel and the wrapped triangles of cheese are ideal as well.

Cottage cheese is also popular, plain or simply mixed with something like chopped pineapple. You could also make a scoopful of cheese into a ball, accompany it with a scoopful of grated apple and raisins, and surround it with a selection of mixed fruit chopped very small. This makes a nutritious, yet delicious, snack that children love.

Green Goddess Dip

Serve this tasty dip surrounded by a selection of raw vegetable sticks, such as carrot, cucumber, red bell pepper, and celery. Add some cherry tomatoes, corn chips, and bread sticks for a nutritious snack.

MAKES 2 ADULT PORTIONS

1 large, ripe avocado
½ tablespoon fresh lemon juice
2 tablespoons cream cheese
1 tablespoon sliced scallion

2 tomatoes, skinned, seeded, and
finely chopped
1 tablespoon diced, red bell pepper
salt and pepper to taste

Cut the avocado in half, pit, and scoop the flesh out of the skin. Mash it together with the rest of the ingredients. This will turn brown if left standing for too long.

Chef's Salad with Turkey and Cheese

MAKES 3 CHILD PORTIONS

Dressing
3 tablespoons light olive oil
1 tablespoon runny honey
1 tablespoon soy sauce
1½ tablespoons freshly squeezed lemon juice

1 Little Gem lettuce, cut into small pieces
2 medium tomatoes (9 oz), skinned,
seeded, and chopped
4½ oz cooked turkey or chicken, diced
⅝ cup Edam cheese, cubed or 1¼ cups
cooked pasta
⅔ cup canned corn kernels

Whisk together all the ingredients for the dressing. Put the rest of the ingredients into a bowl and toss together with the dressing.

Homemade Fast-Food Pizzas

These delicious, easy-to-make pizzas are always popular.

MAKES 4 MINI PIZZAS

1 scallion, finely sliced
4 mushrooms, washed and sliced
1 tablespoon butter
2 tomatoes, skinned, seeded, and chopped
2 teaspoons tomato paste

2 teaspoons basil, chopped
1/3 cup frozen corn kernels
freshly ground black pepper
2 English muffins, split in half
3/8 cup Cheddar cheese, grated

Sauté the scallion and mushrooms in the butter for 2 minutes. Stir in the tomatoes, tomato paste, and basil and cook for 2 more minutes. Cook the corn according to the packet instructions, combine with the tomato mixture, and season with a little black pepper. Toast the split muffins for a few minutes under a hot broiler. Top with the tomato and corn mixture, sprinkle with the grated cheese, and cook under a hot broiler until golden and bubbling.

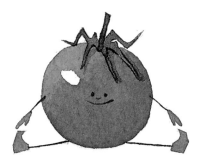

Stuffed Eggs

Cut hard-boiled eggs in half lengthwise and cut a thin sliver off the base of each half so that they stand firm. Fill with finely mashed yolks, mixed with a very small quantity of one of the following:

chopped cucumber, lettuce, tomato, and mayonnaise

OR

cottage cheese and chives

OR

poached salmon and mayonnaise

OR

finely chopped chicken and tomato catsup

OR

canned salmon or tuna, mayonnaise, and chopped scallion

Top-Hat Egg

This is a great snack or breakfast treat for children and they'll have fun helping you to make it. If you wish, sprinkle with grated cheese and pop it under the broiler until golden before serving with a broiled tomato and some sautéed mushrooms.

MAKES 1 ADULT PORTION

1 thick slice of bread
a little butter or margarine

1 egg yolk
salt and pepper

Press out a circle from the center of the bread using a 2-inch-diameter glass. Butter both sides of the bread and fry both pieces for about 1 minute in a small skillet. Flip the bread over, place a small piece of butter in the hole, and let sizzle. Drop the egg yolk into the hole, season lightly, and cook, covered, for about 4 minutes or until set. Serve with the fried circle of bread placed on top of the egg.

On-the-Go Snacks

When you are going on a journey with your toddler, it's a good idea to fill a small plastic container or sandwich bag with a selection of healthy snacks for little fingers to delve into and nibble when they feel hungry.

Fresh fruit like grapes, satsumas, blueberries, bananas, plums, or cherries make an ideal snack for young children. Ready-to-eat dried fruits also make nutritious snacks: for example, mini boxes of raisins, yogurt-coated raisins, apricots, apple rings, mango, dates, figs, prunes, or banana chips.

For something more savory, give mini cheeses, cherry tomatoes, cucumber, or carrot sticks.

You could also offer your child's favorite healthy breakfast cereals, or popcorn, mini rice cakes, or mini sandwiches: for example, Vegemite or peanut butter.

Sandwiches

Sandwiches can come in all shapes and sizes. Try making animal-shaped sandwiches using a cookie cutter. Pinwheel sandwiches are very appealing, too (see page 186).

Toasted sandwiches are a meal in themselves. It is well worth investing in a toasted-sandwich maker, which seals the bread.

Try experimenting with lots of different types of bread: small round pita breads sliced open and stuffed with salad; raisin bread; open sandwiches on soft rolls; bagels (excellent for a toddler to chew on when he is teething); French bread; tortilla wraps; or even a simple sandwich with one side made from white bread and the other brown.

Presentation is very important. A child is far more likely to eat something that looks appealing. Sprinkle the sandwiches with shredded lettuce, or decorate with thinly serrated vegetables, or make your sandwiches into little trains or boats. It doesn't take long and it's fun to do. I think you will find that a lot of toddlers will reach out for your sandwiches.

On the following pages are some suggestions for sandwich fillings. Your toddler will soon let you know his preferences!

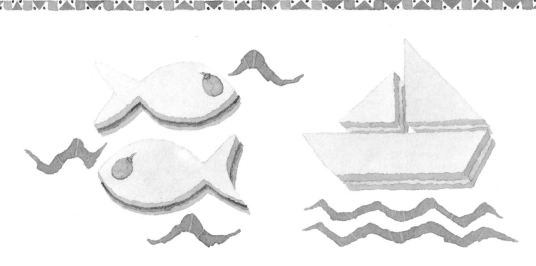

Pinwheel Sandwiches

Remove the crusts from two slices of bread. Place on a board, overlapping the edges slightly, and then roll them together with a rolling pin to join the slices together and gently flatten the bread, making it more pliable. Alternately, cut the crust from the side of a long, rectangular, dense-textured loaf and cut into long, thin slices – this way you can prepare pinwheels without any joins. Spread evenly with butter or margarine and the desired filling and roll up the bread. Cut into slices to make little pinwheels. It is a good idea to prepare these in advance, wrap in plastic wrap, and set aside in the refrigerator – they will slice better if chilled first.

You can even make a variegated pinwheel sandwich by rolling one brown and one white slice of bread (which have both been spread with different but complementary fillings) together.

Chocolate spread and banana
Peanut butter and raspberry jelly
Peanut butter and mashed banana
Cream cheese and ham
Smoked salmon

Peanuts can cause allergic reactions (see page 15)

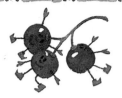

Cream cheese and crushed pineapple (or fruit purée)

Cream cheese, toasted sesame seeds, and mustard and cress

Cream cheese and cucumber

Cream cheese and crushed corn-flakes

Cream cheese in raisin bread with strawberry jelly

Cream cheese in a bagel with slices of smoked salmon

Cream cheese with chopped dried apricots

Cream cheese and redcurrant jelly

Cottage cheese with avocado and lemon juice

Cheese and chutney

Grated cheese and carrot with mayonnaise

Plain ricotta and raisins

Sliced falafel with grated carrot and raisins

Chopped, hard-boiled egg, water-cress, and mayonnaise

Egg mayonnaise with a little curry powder

Chopped, hard-boiled egg with mashed sardines

Tuna mayonnaise and mustard and cress

Tuna or salmon with corn, scal-lion, and mayonnaise

Canned salmon, chopped egg, and mayonnaise

Chopped chicken, mayonnaise, and yogurt with a little curry powder and raisins

Chicken or turkey with chutney

Bacon, lettuce, tomato, and a little mayonnaise

Open Toasted Sandwiches

Toast the bread first, spread with the topping and cook under a hot broiler.

Cheese and tomato

Diced ham and pineapple with grated cheese

Canned sardines in tomato sauce.

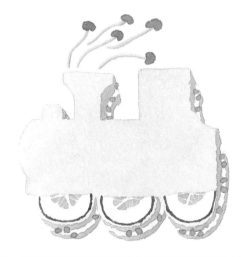

TODDLER MEAL PLANNER

	Breakfast	Lunch	Dinner
Day 1	Fruity Swiss Muesli Yogurt Fruit	Annabel's Juicy Burgers with vegetables Pear, Apple, and Raspberry Crumble with ice cream	Spaghetti with Two-Tomato Sauce Frozen Strawberry-Yogurt Ice Cream
Day 2	Cheese on toast Apricot, Apple, and Pear Custard	Grandma's Tasty Fish Pie Fruit	Chicken Fillets with Mango Chutney and Apricot with vegetables Poached Fruits
Day 3	Oatmeal with honey or jelly Apple purée Petit Suisse	Marinated Chicken on the Griddle with vegetables and French fries Going Bananas	Bow-Ties with Swiss Cheese and Cherry Tomatoes Fruit and ice cream
Day 4	Scrambled eggs Cereal Fruit	Chicken and Apple Balls Snow-Covered Fruit Salad	Nursery Fish Pie Homemade Fruit Gelatin
Day 5	Pineapple and Raisin Muffins Yogurt Fruit	Shepherd's Pie with vegetables Strawberry Rice Pudding	Spaghetti Primavera Fruit
Day 6	Boiled eggs with fingers of toast Prunes Yogurt	Toasted Tuna Muffins Homemade Fruit Gelatin	Bow-Ties with Tomato and Mozzarella Sauce Fruit and ice cream
Day 7	Cereal Cheese Fruit	Chef's Salad with Turkey and Cheese Pear, Apple, and Raspberry Crumble	Tuna Tagliatelle Peaches with Amaretti Biscuits

These meal charts show you how to plan ahead and cook for the whole family together.

FAMILY MEAL PLANNER

	Breakfast	*Lunch*	*Dinner*
Day 1	**Fruity Swiss Muesli** Yogurt	**Annabels' Hidden-Vegetable Tomato Sauce**	**Annabel's Juicy Burgers** with vegetables and potato **Pear, Apple, and Raspberry Crumble** with ice cream
Day 2	**My Favorite Pancakes Apricot, Apple, and Pear Custard**	**Chicken and Apple Balls** and vegetables	**Grandma's Tasty Fish Pie** with vegetables **Snow-Covered Fruit Salad**
Day 3	**French Toast Cutouts** Baked beans	**Tuna and Corn Stuffed Potato** Fruit	**Marinated Chicken on the Griddle** and **Special Fried Rice Frozen Strawberry-Yogurt Ice Cream** or yogurt and fruit
Day 4	Scrambled egg Cereal	**Thai-Style Chicken and Noodles** Fruit salad	**My Favorite Pasta with Broccoli Homemade Fruit Gelatin** and ice cream
Day 5	**Pineapple and Raisin Muffins** Yogurt and honey	**Cod in a Cheese Sauce with Matchstick Vegetables**	**Shepherd's Pie** with vegetables or salad **Poached Fruits**
Day 6	**The Three Bears' Breakfast** Prunes	**Toasted Tuna Muffins** Fruit	**Mini Minute Steaks** with potato **Homemade Fruit Gelatin** and ice cream
Day 7	**Cheese Scramble** and toast Fruit	**Stir-Fried Chicken with Vegetables and Noodles** or **Bar-B-Q Chicken** with vegetables **Going Bananas**	**Gratin of Sole Ratatouille with Rice or Pasta**

INDEX

INDEX

ACKNOWLEDGMENTS

I am indebted to the following people for their help and advice during the writing of this book.

Dr Stephen Herman FRCP, Consultant Pediatrician, Central Middlesex Hospital, London, England.

Margaret Lawson, Senior Lecturer in Pediatric Nutrition, Institute of Child Health, University of London, England.

Professor Charles Brook, Consultant Pediatric Endocrinologist, Middlesex Hospital, London, England.

Dr Sam Tucker FRCP, Consultant Pediatrician, Hillingdon Hospital, London, England.

Jacky Bernett, Community Dietician.

Dr Tim Lobstein, specialist in children's food and nutrition at The London Food Commission.

Carol Nock SRN FCN, Midwife.

Kathy Morgan, State Registered Health Visitor.

My mother, Evelyn Etkind, for all her encouragement in writing this book.

David Karmel, for his patience in teaching me how to use a computer.

Beryl Lewsey for her enthusiasm and hard work.

Ros Edwards, Ian Jackson, Susan Fleming, Fiona Eves and Elaine Partington of Eddison Sadd.

Dr Irving Etkind, for his help in research.

Jane Hamilton, my nanny, for restraining my children from wiping out my manuscript on the computer!

And, most important of all, my husband Simon, my chief guinea pig, for all his support.

THE AUTHOR

Annabel Karmel is a leading author on cooking for children. After the death of her first child, who died of a rare viral disease aged just under three months, Annabel wrote *The Healthy Baby Meal Planner*, which is now an international bestseller. She has written ten other best-selling books including *Superfoods For Babies and Children*, *The Complete First Year Planner* and *Favorite Family Recipes*.

Annabel lives in London and is the mother of three children, Nicholas, Lara, and Scarlett. As a trained cordon bleu cook and young mother, she experienced first-hand the difficulties in feeding young children.

She thoroughly researched all aspects of feeding babies and children to cut through the often confusing and conflicting advice given to parents on the subject. She combined her findings with her own experience and knowledge of cooking, testing each recipe on a panel of babies and toddlers.

Annabel appears frequently on television and writes regularly for magazines and newspapers, including *The Times*, *Practical Parenting*, and *BBC Good Food* magazine. **Visit www.annabelkarmel.com for more recipes and advice.**